ENDOCRINOLOGY RESEARCH AND CLINICAL DEVELOPMENTS

HANDBOOK OF DIABETES FOR GENERAL PRACTITIONERS

ENDOCRINOLOGY RESEARCH AND CLINICAL DEVELOPMENTS

Additional books in this series can be found on Nova's website under the Series tab.

Additional e-books in this series can be found on Nova's website under the e-book tab.

ENDOCRINOLOGY RESEARCH AND CLINICAL DEVELOPMENTS

HANDBOOK OF DIABETES FOR GENERAL PRACTITIONERS

ANIL K. MANDAL
EDITOR

NOVA BIOMEDICAL
New York

Library of Congress Cataloging-in-Publication Data

ISBN: 978-1-63482-821-5
Library of Congress Control Number: 2015942934

Published by Nova Science Publishers, Inc. † New York

This book on Handbook of Diabetes for General Practitioners is dedicated to those individuals who have contributed to make this book into a reality. They are my patients with diabetes; Dr. Moustafa Eldick of Putnam Community Medical Center Palatka, Florida, Nursing Staff of Lakewood Nursing Center, Crescent City. Florida; Janice Pimentel, Tracy Pirtle and Danielle Torrez of Jacksonville Clinic at Saint Augustine, Florida; and Karen Kidwell of Saint Augustine, Florida. Since this book is a product of Mandal Diabetes Research Foundation, dedication extends to Mr. Deepak Singh of New Delhi, India for his interest and support for a joint venture of Harbhajan Singh Diabetes Foundation of India with Mandal Diabetes Research Foundation of USA

Contents

Preface

Diabetes affects people of all ages and races. Diabetes Mellitus (DM) develops because of physiological disturbance of the pancreas, when the organ has a deficient production of insulin. Ancient and medieval medicine understood the disease through symptoms, primarily polyuria and excessive thirst. These symptoms accompanied by appearance of sugar in the urine prompted a diagnosis of DM. DM is the same today as it was centuries ago. The hallmark of DM is hyperglycemia and glycosuria (excessive sugar in blood and urine). Although DM was recognized in 1500 B.C., nothing was done to treat this morbid condition until Frederick Banting identified that DM is caused by a deficiency of insulin. Therefore, the treatment of DM is insulin therapy. Without insulin therapy, high glucose milieu in DM causes severe injury to vascular endothelial cells resulting in the appearance of a gamut of complications including unhealed foot ulcers, gangrene of toes or feet associated with amputation of one or both limbs, acute coronary syndrome and death, blindness, kidney failure, sexual dysfunction and many more. Treating DM with insulin, a replacement therapy, can avert all these complications. But the uniqueness of this therapy is seriously jeopardized by the invasion of commercialism in care of DM. The prevailing commercialism has dictated diabetes care by transforming DM into two types of diabetes, Type 1, insulin deficient, Type 2 insulin resistant. This classification by World Health Organization and American Diabetes Association was orchestrated to help the pharmaceutical industry promote the sale of oral antidiabetic drugs to treat Type 2 DM. Their premise is that metformin is the first line therapy for Type 2 DM, which is prevalent among adults. In author's experience, the majority of adults with DM are insulin deficient requiring insulin for glycemic control. However, a smaller percentage of people with DM is a variant of DM associated with obesity. This variant or Type 2 DM is not the diabetes discovered by Frederick Banting. Thus, on one hand, many adults labeled with Type 2 DM do not have DM. Elevated fasting blood glucose or glycosylated hemoglobin (HbA_1c) is common among people with hypertension and treated with antihypertensive drugs in particular, thiazide diuretics. Doctors, and more often nurse practitioners diagnose them with Type 2 DM and automatically prescribe them metformin and lisinopril. On the other hand, obesity and hyperglycemia can go hand in hand, mainly due to lack of clearance of postprandial hyperglycemia by the muscle. Thus, forced and massive weight reduction induced by bariatric surgery results in remission of hyperglycemia. Their kidney function is normal and the kidney biopsy shows slight or no diabetic change suggesting that hyperglycemia associated with obesity is not DM as described by Frederick Banting. But it is a reversible syndrome of intermediary metabolism. Successive 2-hour postprandial glucose levels or 4-hour oral glucose tolerance test can demonstrate that. Thus, prescription of metformin as a first line therapy in obese individuals with hyperglycemia considered to have Type 2 diabetes is an unjust act. The reason is that overtime beta cell exhaustion induced by metformin could transform this reversible hyperglycemia into a pathological hyperglycemia accompanied by a gamut of microvascular and macrovascular complications over the years. A chapter is included to clarify the issues of obesity and Type 2 DM and how massive weight reduction following bariatric surgery can elucidate the ambiguities.

Some of these issues of prevailing commercialism related to diabetes care have been described in the first book of Diabetes called “Diabetes: A True life story of how to cope and thrive published by Nova Science Publishers Inc. in 2011. This Handbook of Diabetes for General Practitioners” is developed to elaborate on the crossroads in diabetes care and what are the impacts of the crossroads on the vast array of complications that diabetes patients are currently developing. Like the previous book, this current book of diabetes is produced to help patients learn to cope with diabetes and live a complication-free life.

The importance of postprandial hyperglycemia and the relevance of insulin therapy to keep postprandial hyperglycemia under control has been emphasized in this book. Also emphasized in this book is control of hypertension, which is additive to glycemic control by safe anti-hypertensive drugs excluding the use of renin-angiotensin inhibitors drugs. Treatment of diabetes with oral antidiabetic drugs has been excluded in this book. Oral antidiabetic drugs reduce fasting blood glucose but there is no evidence that these drugs reduce the risk of complications. Thus, the intent of the author is to inform the readers of insulin, a replacement therapy for diabetes. Learning of self-care, which is an attribute in effective glycemic control and prevention of complications, has been elaborated in this book. Finally, end stage renal disease (ESRD) and renal replacement therapy (Dialysis) are conventional therapies among diabetic patients; however, they are unconventional in the author's patients. Thus, such a chapter will not be discussed in this book.

Chapter I

Departure from Discovery of Insulin to Save Diabetes Patients from Dying to Treatment with Incretion Therapy to Promote Commercialism

Abstract

Many investigators worked to isolate the internal secretion of the pancreas, which may be insulin, until Frederick Banting prepared the extract in duct-ligated pancreas and succeeded in 1922 in showing that such extract reduced the hyperglycemia and glycosuria in de pancreatized animal prolonged by the repeated injection of alcoholic extract of pancreas. Thus, diabetes mellitus (DM) was defined as a metabolic disorder due to a deficiency of the internal secretion of the pancreas. The main principle of treatment is, therefore to correct the deficiency. If it is found that if a patient is unable to keep sugar-free on a diet compatible with an active useful life, sufficient insulin is administered to meet this requirement since the discovery of insulin in 1922 and commercially available for use in 1923. Millions of patients with DM who developed diabetic comas were saved from dying with insulin treatment. The outcry of the patients with DM has prompted pharmaceutical companies to enhance production of oral antidiabetic agents, which are painless and convenient to take. These drugs lower fasting glucose but do not restore glycemic control; hence do not prevent complications of DM. The classification on of Type 1 and Type 2 DM has resulted in the popularity of idea of oral antidiabetic agents, which have advocated a policy of commercialism and increased the misery of the patients with DM by riddling them with complications.

Introduction and Historical Perspective

(Adapted from Nobel lecture delivered in Stockholm May 26, 1925)

The knowledge that the islets of Langerhans of the pancreas have the function of secreting into the blood of hormone, which plays an essential role in the regulation of the metabolism of carbohydrates, is the outcome of numerous investigations. In 1989, Minkowski and Von Mering discovered the complete extirpation of the pancreas leads to fatal diabetes. Minkowski in his published report in 1893, considered that the antidiabetic function of the pancreas was dependent upon its acting as a ductless gland. Finally, Lagasse and Diamare coined the collection of cells through their work as islets of Langerhans. They concluded that the islets must be responsible for the antidiabetic function. Many investigators worked to isolate the internal secretion of the pancreas, which might be insulin, until Frederick Banting at University of Toronto, Canada prepared the extract in duct-ligated pancreas and succeeded in 1922 in showing that such extract reduced the hyperglycemia and glycosuria in depancreatized dogs. The general symptoms of diabetes such as polyuria and rapid weight loss were alleviated and duration of life of the depancreatized animal was prolonged by the repeated injection of alcoholic extract of pancreas. On the other hand, peculiar symptoms (convulsion and coma) were observed in many of the injected animals, and it was soon possible to show that these were related to the lowering of the blood sugar to very low levels and these symptoms developed when the blood sugar was about 0.045 percent (4.5 mg/dL). Sometimes the animal recovered spontaneously from these symptoms, but more frequently, death occurred. That the lowering of blood sugar is closely related to the occurrence of the symptoms, was proved by the finding that the subcutaneous injection of a solution of glucose was followed, almost immediately, by complete recovery, even in cases in which death was imminent from deep coma. It has been found that glucose is remarkably specific in that regard.

It must be understood that insulin primarily acts by lowering the tension of glucose within the tissue cells, so that the glucose of the blood plasma, with which the tissue glucose is in equilibrium, diffuses into the cells to maintain the tension. By considering the conclusion, it seems justified that the only source from which physiologically effective insulin can be secreted within the animal body is islet tissue

Diabetes and Insulin by Frederick G. Banting, Nobel Lecture Delivered in Stockholm, September 15, 1925

From April 14th in 1921, the pancreas was removed in a number of dogs. The pancreas after removal was found to be shriveled, fibrotic, and about one-third of the original size. The material was tested on a dog rendered diabetic by the removal of the pancreas. Following the intravenous injection, the blood sugar of the depancreatized dogs was reduced to a normal or subnormal level and the urine became sugar-free. Marked improvement was noted in the general condition of the animals as they became stronger and livelier with rapid healing of the wounds and prolongation of the life. The extract was sufficiently purified to be tested on three cases of diabetes mellitus in the wards of Toronto General Hospital. There was a marked reduction in blood sugar and the urine was rendered sugar free.

Thus, diabetes mellitus (DM) was defined as a metabolic disorder due to a deficiency of the internal secretion of the pancreas. The main principle of the treatment is, therefore, to correct the deficiency. If it is found that the patient is unable to keep sugar-free on a diet that compatible with an active, useful life, sufficient insulin is administered to meet this requirement.

In severe cases, insulin was administered subcutaneously three times a day, from one-half to three-quarters of an hour before meals. This was done so that the curve of hypoglycemia produced by the insulin was superimposed on the curve of hyperglycemia produced by the meal. In rare cases, a small fourth dose was given at bedtime to control nocturnal glycosuria. The less severe cases could be satisfactorily treated with a morning and evening dose or a single dose before breakfast. When the insulin treatment was established, if sugar was present in the twenty-four hour urine specimen, the insulin dosage was gradually increased until the patient became sugar-free. If small quantities of urinary sugar persist, it was desirable to find out what period of the day this was excreted. An increase in the dose before the appearance of glycosuria will prevent its occurrence. In severe cases, it was preferable to give the largest dose of insulin in the morning, and reduced doses throughout the day.

Initial Results of Insulin Therapy and Historical Patients Treated with Insulin

On January 11, 1922, the researchers at Toronto General Hospital, Canada were presented with an opportunity to try their pancreatic extract on a 14-year old-child named Leonard Thompson (1908-1935). The young Toronto resident had been diabetic since 1919. He weighed only 65 pounds and was about to slip into a coma. He received the injection of extract prepared by Dr. F Banting and Dr. R Charles Best. The first injection resulted in an allergic reaction. Twelve days later, he was given a second dose further purified by Collip. Thompson's symptoms began to disappear; his blood sugar returned to normal and he was brighter and stronger. He went on to live 13 more years taking doses of insulin. He died at the age of 27 due to diabetic complications. The treatment was quickly promoted and used in a number of distinguished personalities in the scientific community. One of the first people to benefit from the discovery of insulin was treasurer of the Royal College of Physicians of Edinburgh, Sir Norman Purvis Walker (1862-1942) was suffering from diabetes and by 1922, he became emaciated and his colleagues had little hope for his survival. The discoverers of insulin heard of his condition and sent some samples from Canada before it was generally available. When Walker received insulin, the effect was immediate.

An even more significant personality was the spouse of August Krogh (1874-1949) who was awarded Nobel Prize in Physiology or Medicine in 1920. His wife Marie herself was a researcher, and in 1921 she was found to have developed maturity-onset diabetes. While in the USA in November 1922, they were informed that insulin was discovered and purified in Toronto. The couple went to Toronto as guests of John Macleod. Krogh obtained a license for insulin purification. Production was started immediately. The first patient was treated as early as March 13, 1923. Together with the Danish Physician HC Hagedorn Krogh, they founded the Nordic Insulin laboratory. This became the starting point of a very successful Danish pharmaceutical company and research fund. Marie Krogh's diabetes was successfully treated with insulin.

In 1923, Eli Lilly and Co. in Indianapolis started commercial production of insulin, naming their product Isletin Insulin.

Here is an exemplary case report by Banting (summarized):

A 15-year-old female, in the autumn of 1918, developed polyuria and polydipsia and complained of weakness. During the winter, she suffered from pains in the legs and back. In March 1919, these symptoms became worse. The appetite was excessive. She lost much weight. She was placed on diet control. Her condition progressively worsened. On August 16, 1922, she weighed 45 pounds. At this time she was receiving a diet consisting of protein 50g, fat 71 g and carbohydrate 20 g. Insulin treatment was started. The diet was increased to protein 63g, fat 208g, and carbohydrate 97g (2512 calories). Insulin was given 15 to 30 minutes before the morning and evening meals. A sufficient amount of insulin was given to keep the urine free of sugar. Each specimen of urine was examined and the dose of insulin was increased slightly if traces of sugar appeared. When hypoglycemia occurred, orange juice or glucose candy was given. Between August 16, 1922 and January 1, 1923, urine was sugar free except on ten occasions when traces of sugar appeared.

On this treatment, the patient rapidly gained weight from 45 to 105 pounds and felt strong. The diet included foodstuffs such as cereals, bread, potatoes, rice, corn, tapioca, cornstarch, and even honey.

In 1925, she was in the best of her health and expressed in her words "never felt better in all my life."

She had grown four inches and weighed 134 pounds. Her diet consists of carbohydrate 125g, protein 50g, and fat 50g. The insulin required to maintain her urine sugar-free has been reduced about one-third.

Departure from Insulin Treatment to Incretin Therapy in Diabetes Mellitus

Since the discovery of insulin in 1922 and its becoming commercially available for use in 1923, millions of patients with DM who developed diabetic coma were saved from dying with insulin treatment. Many more were saved from developing seriously infected foot ulcers, carbuncles, going blind or undergoing amputation. The outcry of the patients with DM has prompted pharmaceutical companies to enhance production of oral antidiabetic agents. A plethora of agents entered into the market over the years. They lower fasting glucose but do not restore glycemic control because they are not a substitute of insulin. Thus, more DM patients are entering hospitals with severe diabetes complicated by ketoacidosis, renal failure requiring dialysis or presenting with heart attack.

Thus, oral antidiabetic agents have accelerated the business for the professionals and the industry but are not helping the patients to live a good and healthy life.

The latest in the march against insulin treatment is Incretin based therapy. The Incretin (intestinal secretion of insulin) system includes glucose dependent insulintropic polypeptide (previously known as gastric inhibitory polypeptide) and glucagon like peptide -1 (GLP-1)

The system plays an important role in the pathogenesis of Type 2 diabetes, the Incretin effect has mostly been attributed to peptide hormones that are released in the blood stream from intestinal cells in response to a meal. GLP-1, a 30 amino acid peptide is the potent stimulator of oral glucose-induced insulin secretion. GLP-1 controls fasting and postprandial (PP) glucose concentrations mainly by simulating glucose dependent insulin secretion from the beta cells while inhibiting glucagon secretion.

Preparation of Incretin includes GLP-1 receptor agonist and Dipeptidyl peptidase-4 (DPP-4) inhibitors.

GLP-1 receptor agonists called Exenatide sold as Byetta or Victoza and DPP-4 inhibitors includes sitagliptin.

Analysis of Fundamental Problems Related to Oral Antidiabetic Therapy

The classification of Type 1 and Type 2 DM has resulted in the popularity of the idea of oral diabetic agents. Oral antidiabetic agents are not a substitute for insulin, which is the treatment of diabetes mellitus (DM). DM is due to deficiency of insulin, stated in Nobel lecture delivered by Frederick Banting in 1925. Therefore, changing the original definition of DM into Type 1 or Type 2 DM is wrong.

After the introduction of Type 1 or Type 2 DM, Type 2 was the prevalent diabetes in adults totally ignoring the discovery of diabetes and insulin by Banting, Best, Mcleod, and many others in 1922.

The most significant mistake is to label any adult with elevated glucose as Type 2 DM and automatically prescribe metformin. The action surely advocates a policy of commercialism to help pharmaceutical companies to sell their products. Many of these individuals are hypertensive and treated with a thiazide diuretic, which increases glucose mimicking diabetes. Thus, instead of publicizing the epidemic of Type 2 DM, it is important to discontinue thiazide diuretic and repeat laboratory in 2 weeks, and surprisingly blood glucose will be normal. Those with blood glucose of 200mg/dL or more, anytime and not on antihypertensive therapy are likely to have DM as defined by Banting and insulin treatment should be initiated immediately.

Thus, in reality so called Type 2 DM is a misnomer and carries no similarity to the original discovery of diabetes and insulin by Banting, Best, Mcleod and Collip.

References

[1] *History of Diabetes Mellitus.* Editors Savona-Ventura C, Mogensen CE, 2009, Elsevier Masson

[2] Mandal AK, Hiebert LM: Is diuretic-induced hyperglycemia reversible and inconsequential? *J Diab Res Clin Met* 2012; 1:4.

Chapter II

Flaws in Diagnosis of Diabetes and Consequences

Abstract

Diabetes Mellitus or Sugar diabetes or diabetes is common but definitely diabetes, is not epidemic. Publicity of the epidemic of diabetes comes from the wrong diagnosis. Putting a label of Type 2 diabetes on someone having elevated fasting blood glucose (FBG)> 126 mg/dL (> 7 mmol/L) is wrong. Elevated FBG is very commonly due to antihypertensive drug therapy including beta-blocker, calcium channel blocker and most commonly a thiazide diuretic, hydrochlorothiazide or chlorthalidone. Thus, the first step will be to temporarily discontinue the blood pressure lowering drug and repeat the basic metabolic panel in the fasting and 2-h postmeal period in 2 weeks. Thus, initial diagnosis of Type 2 diabetes or diabetes will be disproved by decreased glucose levels in the repeat testing. Hence, it is a mistake to prescribe oral antidiabetic agents to someone without a proven diagnosis of diabetes. It is important to remember that many complications of diabetes that emerge in the course of time are due to wrong diagnosis of diabetes at the first step.

Introduction

Diabetes Mellitus (DM) is a metabolic disease characterized by hyperglycemia (high glucose level in the blood) and glucosuria (variable amount of glucose in the urine) and is due to deficiency in insulin secretion from the pancreas [1].

This chronic hyperglycemia is associated with long term damage, dysfunction, and failure of various organs, especially the eyes, kidneys, nerves, heart and blood vessels [2]. DM remains undiagnosed for a long time especially in middle aged or elderly subjects because hyperglycemia manifests soberly in older age groups. In children or young adults, hyperglycemia gives rise to explosive symptoms such as polyuria, polydipsia and rapid weight loss which force family to seek medical advice and result in diagnosis of DM. On the contrary, adults seek medical advice for retention of urine (neurogenic bladder), erectile dysfunction, chest pain, or decreased vision and are found to have DM for the first time. Interestingly more and more adults are being transported into the emergency room of local hospitals in poor condition and they are found to have diabetic ketoacidosis, infected foot ulcer, gangrenous foot or toes, or severe renal failure. Many adults with diabetes have symptoms like polyuria, nocturia and polydipsia but of lesser severity and were ignored mainly because they don't have health insurance and have no means to pay doctor's office visit.

On the other hand, those who felt that these symptoms are warning signs of diabetes went to a family health clinic where they have received a diagnosis of Type 2 DM and an automatic prescription of metformin and Lisinopril. In the course of time, some of them have developed one or more complications as stated above and then received a prescription of insulin therapy. But it is too late to start treatment with insulin, in which the patient is deficient. The damage to organs caused by high glucose has already set in.

The delay in diagnosis and appropriate treatment of diabetes are mainly due to the gaps in knowledge among the professionals, too much weight put on DM Type 1 and Type 2 classification, and total reliance on glycosylated hemoglobin (HbA1c) to assess glycemic control. According to the World Health Organization, Type 1 DM encompasses the vast majority of cases that are primarily due to pancreatic islet beta cell destruction and that are prone to develop ketoacidosis. This form includes both children and an unspecified number of adults. The class Type 2 DM includes the most prevalent form of DM. Patient with this form of DM are generally overweight or obese and associated with high insulin or insulin resistance.

Analysis of Pitfalls of Diabetes Classification

1. Beta cell destruction is an anatomical finding. There is no clinical method to identify this anatomical finding, but it is manifested by insulin deficiency. Thus, patients must be treated with insulin replacement. Hence, why not use the past terminology insulin-dependent diabetes.
2. Ketoacidosis is a component of Type 1 DM and is commonly seen in children. Currently many adults are admitted into hospitals with a diagnosis of diabetic ketoacidosis. Why do these adults develop ketoacidosis? Because they have no health insurance or lost their health insurance, and thus they could not afford to take insulin - again insulin deficiency. What is the difference in diabetic ketoacidosis between children and adults? Both age groups are insulin deficient.
3. The vast majority of patients treated in the office have their FBG and 2hPPG out of range despite insulin therapy because of non-compliance in diet. Hypoglycemic peaks caused by insulin therapy falls short of hyperglycemic peaks produced by big meals.
4. Very few diabetes subjects are obese and these diabetes subjects show sustained hyperglycemia despite high insulin therapy; we might call this insulin resistant diabetes or metabolic syndrome.

Logistic Approach to Diagnosis and Risk Analysis

Control of Diabetes and Prevention of Its Complications

While untreated hyperglycemia, or uncontrolled hyperglycemia but treated with one or more oral agents, is associated with a high risk to develop one or more microvascular complications, treatment of diabetes with insulin generally affords protection from microvascular complications. The most common practice to assess glycemic control is through HbA1c because it is a convenient test and universally available. However, there is very little information available with regard to the relationship of glycemic control using HbA1c and outcome measures. Most outcome measures, especially cardiovascular outcomes, have been related to post challenge or postprandial hyperglycemia. Here is an example to that effect.

Decode study group has shown that the risk for cardiovascular death increases threefold as 2-hour post challenge glucose levels increase from 54 to 199 mg/dL, although these levels are all in the non diabetic range. Data were adjusted for age, gender, weight, systolic blood pressure, cholesterol and smoking during the 11 years of follow-up for the 29,714 patients in the Diabetes Epidemiology Collaborative Analysis of Diagnostic Criteria in Europe [2].

Cardiovascular disorders are common in diabetes and most other studies like Decode have shown that 2PPG above 200mg/dL (> 11.1 mmol/L) is associated with a high risk of mortality [3].

Renally, we have shown that renal function sharply decreases with elevation of glucose at 2hPP period <200> 200 mg/dL. Even though we did not find a significant difference in serum creatinine or eGFR between 2hPPG <200mg/dL> 200 mg/dL, by innovating the factor of d (2hPPG-FBG) we found significant elevation of serum creatinine or a decrease of eGFR with 2 hPPG above 200mg/dL [4] Postprandial hyperglycemia has been reported by numerous authors as a critical factor in diabetic complications [5].

Despite prevailing information about the importance of 2hPPG in diabetes care, providers are educated to order HbA1c every 3 months to assess glycemic control. Here again comes the commercial interest as a guiding principle in diabetes care. Most oral antidiabetic agents reduce HbA1c, for instance from 8 to 7%, an effect that makes providers happy that their patients are doing well, and creates jubilation for the pharmaceutical companies. However, this joy or jubilation is artificial because no correlation is found between HbA1c and renal function tests. There may be good correlation between FBG, 2hPPG, and HbA1c, but renal function deteriorates as a result of uncontrolled postprandial hyperglycemia [6].

Hindrances to Effective Control of Diabetes Mellitus

It is imperative that we strive for early detection and treatment of DM, so that complications may be averted. Treatment of diabetes and its complications are costly, for instance chronic kidney disease. Here is the cost analysis from Medicare from 1993 to 2011 showing progressive increase in the cost of caring for DM. This may be mainly due to treatment of its complication.

One such example is chronic kidney disease (CKD), shown below.

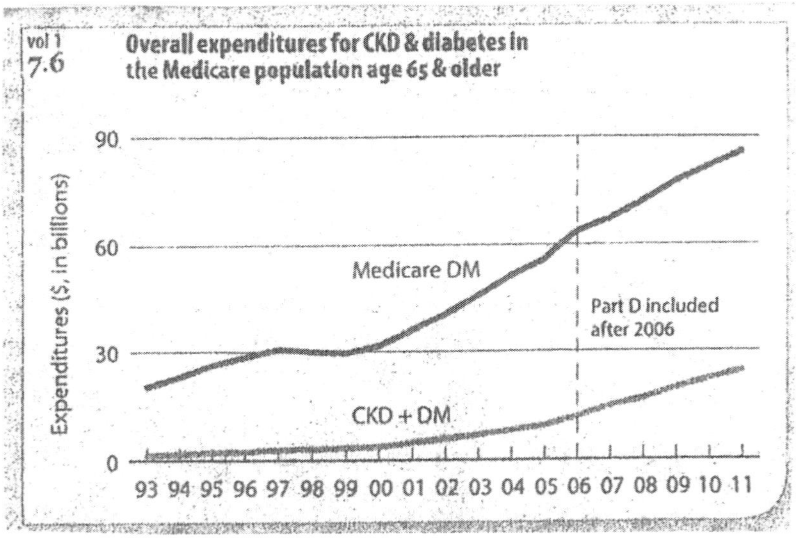

Notwithstanding increasing awareness, adequate funding for diabetes research and a plethora of oral antidiabetic medication to treat diabetes, complication rates including amputation and end stage renal disease are on the rise. The Los Angeles Times as of March 2009 reported "Over the last 15 years the US rate of foot amputations from complications of diabetes has soared, approaching 100,000 annually, according to studies and Government Statistics."

All these complications are due to inappropriate diagnosis and inadequate therapy. What can be done to increase the solidarity of appropriate diagnosis of diabetes and initiation of appropriate therapy? The following approaches are proposed to improve the diagnosis. It is time-consuming but must be done.

Here is an example of fallacy of diagnosis of diabetes.

1. Patient has a fasting basic metabolic panel (BMP) drawn
   Glucose: 140mg/dL (7.7 mmol/L)
   Diagnosis: Diabetes
   Fallacy: 1) Sensitivity 31%
   2) Specificity 100%

The test is not sensitive because this elevated glucose could not be due to other causes. The most common cause of elevated FBG is a thiazide diuretic (hydrochlorothiazide, chlorthalidone or metolazone) These diuretics alone or in combination with a loop diuretic such as furosemide, bumetanide or torsemide increase FBG as high as 200mg/dL or even higher mimicking severe diabetes. Whether any of the diuretics increase 2hPPG is unknown for the simple reason that the 2hPP basic metabolic panel is rarely ordered. Therefore, this lack of information is due to lack of knowledge among professionals.

Here is a great example of this fallacy.

A 70 y white female was first seen in the office on June 9, 2014 with a long history of hypertension, and diabetes for less than 1 year. Medication at this visit includes metformin 500mg PO AM and PM, diltiazem 240mg P.O daily and metoprolol ER 50mg AM and PM. The focus here is about diabetes. Author has raised the question, does she have diabetes? Her serial FBG, 2hPPG, HbA1c, and medication is presented in Table 1. From Table 1 it should be noted that glucose levels increased after discontinuation of metformin; 2hPPG higher than FBG. However, both FBG and 2hPPG reach their highest levels on July 14th after initiation of chlorthalidone and spironolactone.

Table 1.

2014 Date	FBG (mg/dL)	2hPPG (mg/dL)	HbA1c (%)	Medications
June 9	134	NA	NA	Metformin 500mg 1x twice a day Diltiazem 240mg 1 x once a day Metoprolol ER 500mg 1 x twice a day
Metformin discontinued				
June 16	151	186	6.4	Added Chlorthalidone 50 mg daily Spironolactone 50 mg 1 x three a day
June 23	140	164	NA	Increase Spironolactone 50mg q 6h
July 7	162	186	6.3	Chlorthalidone 50mg daily Reduced Spironolactone 25mg 1x TID
July 14	177	207	6.7	Metroprolol 50mg daily Spironolactone 25mg TID Amlodipine 10mg 1 x daily Chlorthalidone 25mg M-W-F
Aug 14	140	128		

NA= not applicable.

However, after reducing chlorthalidone and spironolactone, both FBG and 2hPPG decreased, FBG was slightly elevated suggesting diabetes but normal 2hPPG refutes diabetes. A group of investigators from Italy studied the outcome of new-onset diabetes in treated hypertensive subjects compared to those with previously known diabetes. They found that subjects in whom diabetes developed were exposed to diuretics, calcium channel blockers and angiotensin converting enzyme inhibitors more frequently than in those in whom diabetes did not develop [7].

Steps to Be Taken to Avoid any Error in Diagnosis and Treatment of Diabetes

1. It is a serious mistake to put a label of diabetes or Type 2 diabetes on anyone with elevated blood glucose levels at the first instance.
2. Take time to check all medicines. Very commonly, patients may be taking a beta blocker or a thiazide diuretic for treatment of hypertension. Hypertension is much more prevalent than diabetes.
3. In case of the above, we must temporarily discontinue beta blocker or thiazide diuretic for 2 weeks and repeat FBG and 2hPPG after 2 weeks. The dilemma will be settled if both glucose levels are normal or elevated FBG but normal 2hPPG, as in Table 1
4. Repeat BMP with fasting and 2hPPG after 4 weeks. Results may be clearer for or against the diagnosis of diabetes. Both will be greatly elevated in case of established diabetes.
5. You may order HbA1c but it will add nothing to the diagnosis because it will be elevated whether caused by a beta blocker or a diuretic as in Table 1. However, it will be much higher in established diabetes.
6. Avoid labeling Type 1 or Type 2 diabetes. This classification adds nothing to diabetes care. Just say you have diabetes or no diabetes as determined by 2h-PPG.
7. Remember anybody with established diabetes has a high risk of developing complications if not treated with insulin.

References

[1] Frederick Banting: Diabetes and Insulin Nobel Prize Speech delivered in Stockholm, September 15, 1925.

[2] Decode study Group: Is the current definition of diabetes relevant to mortality risk from all causes and cardiovascular and non-cardiovascular disease? *Diabetes Care* 2003; 26: 288-696.

[3] Aryangat AV, Gerich JE, Type 2 diabetes: Postprandial hyperglycemia and increased cardiovascular risk. Vasc Health and Risk Management 2010; 6: 145-155.

[4] Mandal, AK. Hiebert LM, Khamis H. dglucose is linked to renal function changes in diabetes. *Diab Res Clin Pract* 2011; 91: 190-194.

[5] Gerich JE. Clinical significance, pathogenesis and management of postprandial hyperglycemia. *Arch Intern Med* 2003; 163:1306-1316.

[6] Nosadini R, Tonolo G. Relationship between blood glucose control, pathogenesis and progression of diabetic nephropathy. *J Am Soc. Nephrol* 2004; 15 (Suppl 1) : S1-S5.

[7] Verdeachia P, Reboldi G, Angeli F, Borgionic C, Gattobigio R, Filipucci L et al. Adverse prognostic significance of onset diabetes in treated hypertensive subjects. *Hypertension* 2004; 43: 963-9.

Chapter III

Prevailing Commercialism in Diabetes Care Is the Road to Diabetes Complications

Abstract

Diabetes is the greatest challenge in medical practice; some or many of the problems like heart failure, renal failure, urinary retention, or recurrent vomiting may be related to diabetes. The focus of this chapter is to alert the professionals to be serious in ordering appropriate tests to document diabetes mellitus (DM). DM is a poor man's disease; many do not know they have DM until complications show up such as urinary retention, foot ulcer or chest pain associated with acute coronary syndrome. These people are ordered to go to doctors' offices or the emergency room of a local hospital. But the nuisance of the current practice of diabetes is the diagnosis of Type 2 diabetes in any adult person with slightly elevated fasting blood (FBG), for example 140mg/dL (7.7 mmol/L) and an automatic prescription of metformin and Lisinopril. The provider did not know that the patient was taking hydrochlorothiazide, which will increase FBG mimicking DM. Similarly, a person might have been working under the hot sun and gotten dehydrated resulting in hypokalemia and elevated FBG.

Therefore, the professionals must be aware of the history of the patients medications, which may be diabetogenic such as diuretics, immune suppressive drugs such as tacrolimus, sirolimus and must refrain from prescribing metformin and Lisinopril, thus increasing the risk of acute or chronic renal failure. For any questions in the diagnosis of DM, it is important to order 2-h basic metabolic panel (BMP) after breakfast or lunch, and glucose levels of > 200mg/dL (11.1 mmol/L) confirm the diagnosis of diabetes. Blood glucose of less than 200mg/dL may be suspicious of DM and requires repetition of BMP in 3 months. Similarly, when diagnosis of DM is confirmed, the recommended therapy is insulin, details of which will be found in the text. Metformin may be used as a supplement to insulin but not as substitute for insulin and a prescription of Lisinopril is a call for end-stage renal disease and dialysis. Hence, a prescription of Lisinopril must be avoided.

Diuretic Is a Common Cause of Hyperglycemia Mimicking Diabetes

Diabetes Mellitus (DM) or diabetes, will be interchangeably used throughout the book. Diabetes is the greatest challenge in medical practice; some or many of the problems the patients brings to doctors' offices or to the hospitals are often related to diabetes. Diabetes is a lifelong disease producing much physical and emotional strain on the family and the treatment of its complications is producing a large economic burden on the healthcare system. Diabetes per se is easy to treat but not the complications, which are on the rise. The latter is mainly due to intervention of commercialism in every step of diabetes care. The adverse effect of commercialism intervening diabetes care is mainly due to profound gaps in the knowledge of the professionals who are labeling all adults with elevated blood glucose as having Type 2 DM, and handling over automatic prescriptions of metformin and Lisinopril. A plethora of oral antidiabetic agents are available and they are convenient to take, Inappropriate recommendations of angiotensin converting enzyme inhibitor (ACEI) and or angiotensin receptor blocker (ARB) as renoprotective drugs in diabetes have paved the road to diabetes complications.

Diabetes is a poor man's disease; hence many patients with diabetes cannot afford to see a doctor. They are generally treated by a nurse practitioner or a physician's assistant in a free health clinic or brought into hospital emergency room when they are sick with ketoacidosis or unhealed and infected foot ulcer. In doctors' offices or community health clinics people with slightly elevated fasting blood glucose (FBG) for example, 140mg/dl (7.7 mmol/L) or glycosylated hemoglobin (HbA1c) > 6.5% are immediately diagnosed to have type 2 DM. Professionals most likely do not know that the elevated FBG or HbA1c may be due to hypertensive therapy such as hydrochlorothiazide (HCTZ) or chlorthalidone, which is most commonly prescribed for the treatment of hypertension. More people have hypertension than diabetes. Thus, the patients in question here are hypertensive and treated with the above drug. Thus, the most appropriate measures would be to hold the drugs for 2 weeks and repeat the laboratory to confirm if indeed the elevated glucose was drug-induced or due to diabetes. Here is an example to illustrate the dilemma.

A 69-year-old white male makes a regular visit to a Hypertension clinic on July 7, 1993. He was taking a combination of HCTZ 25mg and triamterene (K-retaining agent) 37.5mg (maxzide ® 25) daily and nifedipine 10mg P.O. three times daily. Renal function panel (Fasting) done on July 7 showed markedly elevated glucose. A question of type 2 DM was raised by the nurse practitioner in the clinic. A spot urine test for electrolytes and creatinine was ordered. Maxzide was discontinued and a repeat renal function panel was ordered in 2 weeks. The results are shown in Table 1.

Table 1.

1993	July 7	July 21
Glucose (mg/dL)	200	105
BUN (mg/dL)	30	19
Serum Cr (mg/dl)	2.1	1.7
Na (mmol/L)	140	143
K (mmol/L)	3.7	3.9
Chloride (mmol/L)	104	107
CO2 (mmol;/L)	26	28
Spot Urine Values		
Na (mmol/L)	37.4	86.5
Cr (mg/dL)	165	149.4
Cr= creatinine		

Thus, marked hyperglycemia mimicking diabetes was clearly due to volume depletion caused by hydrochlorothiazide. Low Urinary Na and low kidney function before, and increase in urinary Na and improvement in kidney function after discontinuation of HCTZ, is supportive evidence of volume depletion. Low K of 3.7 impairs insulin release and causes hyperglycemia. A nurse practitioner attempted to prescribe him metformin but was stopped by the author. New onset diabetes mellitus induced by diuretic has been described by the author [1].

Diuretics are very commonly used drugs in medical practice for the treatment of hypertension, congestive heart failure, or edematous disorders. Therefore, innumerable patients like this patient will show elevated blood glucose or HbA1c and are likely to be diagnosed as having Type 2 diabetes and started on metformin and Lisinopril. Thus, the epidemic of Type 2 DM described in news media or medical journals is untrue and unfounded and is mainly due to gaps in knowledge of the professionals. The gaps in knowledge of the professionals have permitted the pharmaceutical industry to capture a big market for the sale of the drugs, which may not have any effect of protection like insulin against diabetes complications. The result is progressive worsening of diabetes and onset of acute renal failure or slowly progressive chronic renal failure [2].

Definition and Caveat of Classification of Diabetes

The fact remains that many patients do not know what "Type 2 DM" means. Even a vast majority of professionals don't know the definition of Type 1 and Type 2 DM. Most professionals act like "birds" repeating the words Type 1 and Type 2 DM by hearing from other people. In most or all journals with published articles on diabetes the very same thing is noted; patients with Type 1 and Type 2 DM with no explanations of how they came up with these diagnoses. Very few professionals have the curiosity or courage to ask others what is meant by Type 2 DM. Patients are afraid to ask doctors for explanations. According to the World Health Organization (WHO) adults with diabetes tend to have high insulin or ineffective insulin whereas childhood diabetes is associated with insulin deficiency. However, it seems that these classifications of Type 1 and Type 2 DM were made to help the pharmaceutical industry popularize these oral agents, which are most convenient to take, thus undermining use of insulin. This classification of Type 1 and Type 2 DM is considered not tenable in the current practice of diabetes.

An increasing number of adults are seen in the emergency room of hospitals presenting with features like polyuria, polydipsia or ketoacidosis mimicking Type 1 DM. Some already have established diabetes but developed ketoacidosis because they don't have health insurance and could not afford to buy insulin, hence they remained untreated. Some are newly diagnosed diabetes with random glucose ranging from 300 to 400mg/dL, requiring hospital admission for glycemic control. Much emphasis is laid upon glycosylated hemoglobin (HbA1c) to determine the severity of diabetes and the effectiveness of therapy in attaining glycemic control. Sure enough, previously developed oral antidiabetic agents and many new emerging ones reduce HbA1c more than insulin. In an unpublished study from India, mean pre-treatment Hba1c was 7.03% and after 15 months of metformin treatment, HbA1c decreased to mean 6.9%, a finding that has increased the reputation of metformin as the drug of choice for diabetes. Compared to this enlightened finding, metformin has minimal effect in lowering 2-hPPG. Numerous studies have confirmed that postprandial hyperglycemia is critical to diabetes complications in particular cardiovascular disorders and cardiovascular death [3]. There is little or no information concerning the renal effect of postprandial hyperglycemia. Our observation affirms that uncontrolled postprandial hyperglycemia is associated with foot ulcers, gangrene, and renal failure [4].

Oral Antidiabetic Therapy

In the past, children were brought into doctors' offices for polyuria; excessive thirst and rapid weight loss and they were diagnosed as having Type 1 DM and started on insulin therapy. Now many adults present with the same symptoms and were found to have uncontrolled diabetes but because of prevailing commercialism, they are prescribed metformin, glyburide and Lisinopril instead of insulin. The subtle difference between children and adults is that children almost invariably develop symptoms of diabetes but adults often don't. Adults may not manifest the disease until an organ is damaged. Some of the symptoms for which adults often visit doctors' offices or hospitals include urinary retention due to neurogenic bladder, sexual frigidity/dysfunction, unhealed and infected foot ulcers, or gangrene. In fact, diabetes is often detected for the first time in patients brought into emergency of a local hospital for chest pain [4].

After having the above background it is not understood why we still use Type 1 and Type 2 diabetes classification. How can one differentiate who has what type of diabetes? Why can we not make things simple: just say you have diabetes or you don't. What does this classification add in diabetes care? Obese people have impaired glucose tolerance and have different diabetes.

Diabetes is defined by elevation of blood glucose higher than 200mg/dL. (>11.1 mmol/L) in a post-meal glucose challenge or oral glucose tolerance test [5].

There is no consensus in the application of FBG, 2hPPG, or HbA1c in glycemic control [6]. An important reason for lack of consensus is to popularize HbA1c as a surrogate of glycemic control because HbA1c is reduced by almost all oral agents [7]. Thus, the main purpose in diabetes care is the underlying commercialism to help pharmaceutical companies sell a plethora of oral agents.

There is no evidence in the literature allowing the professionals to inform patients that these drugs are beneficial in terms of outcome measures such as prevention of heart attack or end stage renal disease or improvement in erectile function.

Occasional studies showed that the use of metformin alone or metformin in combination with insulin in Type 2 diabetes reduced the risk of myocardial infraction [8] However, this finding was refuted by another study wherein 390 patients treated with insulin were assigned to randomly receive metformin or a placebo. The primary endpoints were aggregate of mortality. Metformin improved glycemic control and reduced insulin requirements but did not reduce the primary endpoint [9].

There was no study ever done with head to head comparison between insulin and oral antidiabetic agents on a long-term basis in answering the protection for outcome measures. However, a few studies including diabetes control and complications trial research group showed that intensified insulin therapy retards the microvascular complications of diabetes [10, 11].

Authors' own patients are treated with a combination of Glargine (Lantus®) or detemir (Levemir®) after breakfast and dinner (12 h apart) and fast acting insulin (aspart), Novolin® or Humulin® before each meal and at bedtime. Those who still show 2hPPG above 200mg/ dL (> 11.1 mmol/L) take additional regular insulin or fast acting insulin post meal according to a standard or high dose sliding scale if kidney function is normal. Low dose sliding scale is recommended if kidney function is reduced. Those who are diet non-compliant and still show 2hPPG in excess of 200mg/dL receive alpha-glycosidase inhibitors such as acarbose 50mg or 100mg with each meal. These drugs interfere with hydrolysis of carbohydrates and delay absorption of monosaccharides. This drug must be taken with meals to lower 2hPPG level. This paradigm of therapy has made author's patients live a complication free life. Thus, the most important aspect of management of diabetes is to focus on prevention of complications. In primary care or endocrinology practices, most commonly HbA1c is ordered to determine glycemic control. There is nothing wrong in doing that but its correlation with outcome measures such as cardiovascular disorder (CVD) or renal failure is poor. Interestingly, 2hPPG is seldom ordered by primary care physicians or endocrinologists. It is possible that they may be unaware of the importance of 2hPPG or postprandial hyperglycemia. In order to make a correct diagnosis of diabetes and determine its severity one must order a test, which has the highest sensitivity and specificity. 2h post challenge glucose > 200 mg/dL has 97% sensitivity, 100% specificity, and 100% positive predictive value for the diagnosis of diabetes. FBG of 140mg/dL (7.7 mmol/L) has 31% sensitivity, although it has 100% positive predictive value [5].

Postprandial Hyperglycemia

In diabetes, the postprandial phase is characterized by a rapid and large increase in blood glucose levels. The possibility that the post prandial "hyperglycemic spikes" may be relevant to the onset of cardiovascular complications has received much attention. Epidemiological studies and preliminary intervention studies have shown that postprandial hyperglycemia is a direct and independent risk factor for cardiovascular disorder [12]. A consisted body of data demonstrates a robust association between postprandial glucose levels and cardiovascular risk. Large epidemiological studies have shown a continuous graded relationship between the level of post glucose challenge glycemia and the risk for events including coronary heart disease, stroke, sudden cardiac death, and peripheral vascular disease [13].

Besides Cardiovascular disorder, evidence is meager with regard to the relationship between post-prandial hyperglycemia and other diabetic complications, such as nephropathy. However, our own studies have shed some light in defining the relationship of postprandial hyperglycemia to renal function changes. To obviate the dilemma about the superiority between FBG and 2hPPG, we have innovated dglucose (2hPPG-FBG) and related dglucose to renal function changes in 56 patients with established diabetes. We found a statistically significant negative correlation between dglucose and eGFR in those who had 2h-PPG more than 200mg/dL. In patients whose 2hPPG was higher than 200mg/dL, for every 100mg/dL increase in dglucose, d (2hPP-F) serum creatinine increases by 0.11 mg/dL and deGFR decreases by 3.73

ml/min, while in patients whose 2hPP glucose is less than 200mg/dL, for every 100mg/dL increase in dglucose little change is seen in dScr or deGFR [14].

Thus, data from older and relatively newer literature agree that postprandial hyperglycemia should be detected, monitored, and treated aggressively with the paradigm of insulin therapy already stated [14].

Finally, we have convincingly demonstrated that postprandial hyperglycemia reduces renal function. Other authors in the past stated that long-term glycemic control through mealtime abnormality represents a promising means of early therapeutic intervention, and thus for the prevention of progression to renal disease [15].

References

[1] Mandal AK, Heibert LM. Is diuretic-induced hyperglycemia reversible and inconsequential. *J Diab Res Clin Met* 2012; 1:4.

[2] Mandal AK, Hiebert LM: Renal protection in diabetes: Is it affected by glucose control or inhibition of renin-angiotensin pathway. *Clin Nephrol* 2008: 69: 169-178.

[3] Gerich JE. Post prandial hyperglycemia and cardiovascular disease. *Endo Pract* 2006; 12 (Suppl) 47-51.

[4] Mandal AK, Hibert LM: Diabetes Mellitus: Too many controversies affecting care. *J US-China Med Scie* 2013: 10: 121-127.

[5] Harris MI: Undiagnosed NIDDM, clinical and public health issues. *Diabetes Care* 1993; 16: -642-652.

[6] Mandal AK, Hiebert LM: Dilemma in diabetes relates to its complications strategies for prevention. *J DiabRes Clin met* 2012; 11.

[7] Liu SC, Tu YK, Chine MN, Chien KL: Effect of antidiabetic agents added to metformin on glycemic control, hyperglycemia and weight change in patients with type diabetes network meta-analysis. *Diab Obese Metab* 2012; 14: 810-20.

[8] Holman RR, Pal SK, Bethel MA, Mathews DR, Neil. A 10-year follow-up of intensive glucose control in Type 2 diabetes. *N Engl J Med* 2008; 359: 577-589.

[9] Kooy A, deJager J, Hehert P, Bets D, Wilffele MG, Donker AJM, et al. Long term effects of metformin on metabolism and microvascular and macrovascular disease in patients with Type 2 diabetes mellitus. *Arch Intern Med* 2009; 169: 616-625.

[10] Reichard P, Berglyria B, Britz A, Car I, Nilsson BY, Rosen Q Vist U, Intensified conventional Insulin treatment regards the complications of diabetes. The SDIS (Stockholm Diabetes Intervention Study) after 5 years. *J Intern Med* 1991; 23:101-108.

[11] The diabetes control and complications trial research group: The effect of intensive treatment of diabetes on the development and progression of long-term complications in insulin dependent diabetes mellitus. *N Engl J Med* 1993; 329:977-986.

[12] Cavalot F, Petrelli A, Traversa M, Bonomo K, Fiora E, Conte M, Antossi G, Costa G. Trovati M. Postprandial blood glucose is a stronger predictor of cardiovascular events than fasting glucose in Type 2 diabetes Mellitus. *J Clin Endocrinol Met* 2006; 91: 813-9.

[13] DECODE study group. Is the current definition of diabetes relevant to mortality risk from all causes and cardiovascular and non-cardiovascular diseases. *Diabetes care* 2003; 26: 688-96.

[14] Mandal AK, Hiebert LM, Khamis H, dglucose is linked to renal function changes in diabetes. *Diab Res Clin Pract* 2011; 91: 190-194.

[15] Feldt-Rasmussen B. Postprandial hyperglycemia: Potential relationship to the development and progression of diabetic nephropathy. *Diab Obesity and Metabolism 2000*; 2 (Suppl1): S13-20.

Chapter IV

Complications of Diabetes

Abstract

Complications of diabetes are numerous and by themselves make a separate textbook of diabetes. Unfortunately, most of the complications of diabetes are due to misdiagnosis of diabetes, preponderant use of oral antidiabetic drugs to treat diabetes, and scarce use of insulin or late use of insulin when complications have set in, such as foot ulcers or renal failure.

A prevalent complication of diabetes is end stage renal disease (ESRD) developing as a result of non-insulin treatment of diabetes accompanied by aggressive therapy with angiotensin converting enzyme inhibitor (ACEI) and or angiotensin receptor blockers (ARB). ESRD requiring dialysis has imposed a serious economic burden on Medicare or other insurances and on the families in the countries where dialysis is not paid by health insurances.

Thus, the truthful intention of diabetes care is to treat diabetes with insulin to reduce the risk of ESRD and minimizing the need for dialysis therapy. Educating the patients to take responsibility for their illness, with diet control, taking insulin, and keeping feet clean and dry is an integral part of prevention strategy of diabetic complications.

Introductory to Complications of Diabetes

People with diabetes are often riddled with a variety of complications. Patients with one complication, for instance unhealed foot ulcers, urinary retention or erectile dysfunction are often found to have additional complications upon examination. An accompaniment of a major complication, which made the patient to visit a doctor office is protein in the urine or decreased kidney function. Before going any further on this discussion, let us ask some fundamental questions about complications. These questions are

1. Why do diabetes subjects develop complications?
2. Does high glucose alone give rise to complications?
3. Is current therapy for diabetes than the disease itself more responsible for the complications?

Answers to these questions will be found in a composite fashion but not necessarily in an individual fashion.

Type of Diabetic Complications

Two types of complications are seen among diabetes subjects.

A. Acute complications
B. Chronic complications

A. Acute Complications

Acute complications encompass markedly elevated glucose associated with fluid, electrolytes, and acid base disorders giving rise to what is called diabetic ketoacidosis. Markedly elevated glucose, for instance above 200 mg/dL (above 11.1 mmol/L), in a sustained fashion for days or a month results in profound loss of fluid and electrolytes as a results of osmotic diuresis from glycosuria associated with uncontrolled hyperglycemia.

Diabetic Ketoacidosis (DKA) is a common complication being increasingly found in adults with diabetes. These patients are brought into the hospital in poor mental state and with severe dehydration. Omission of insulin is the most common precipitant of DKA [1] Other contributing factors for DKA include infection, stress of surgical procedures and cardiovascular disorders such as myocardial infarction or stroke. These factors cause more dehydration and increase in insulin counter-regulatory hormones and worsening of peripheral insulin resistance. Medications such as diuretics, beta-blockers, corticosteroids, antipsychotics and/or anticonvulsants may affect carbohydrates metabolism and volume status and therefore, could precipitate DKA.

Due to increased lipolysis and decreased lipogenesis, abundant free fatty acids are converted to ketone bodies: beta hydroxybutyrate and acetoacetate. Hyponatremia and hypokalemia are common. Renal function decreases due to hypovolemia. Because of reduced kidney function, serum K may be normal initially but patients with DKA are fundamentally hypokalemic. Severe hypophosphatemia is common during and after treatment with insulin. Normal saline infusion and intravenous drip of insulin as per institutional protocol are the mainstay of therapy. Electrolyte disorders are reversible but require intensive replacement therapy and monitoring by physicians knowledgeable in the area.

B. Chronic Complications

Many chronic complications are observed in people with diabetes. Chronic complications vary with age, gender, race, social and economic conditions, access to health care facility and most importantly, motivation of the patients themselves to stay healthy.

Numerically chronic complications comprise unhealed foot ulcer, gangrene of one or more toes, amputation, erectile dysfunction, renal failure, retinopathy with decreased vision, urinary retention, diarrhea or vomiting and dementia. While all of these complications are attributed to no use of insulin therapy, non-compliance in diet and attitude of self-destruction are pivotally important. Inadequate treatment refers to treatment with only oral antidiabetic agents or with miniscule doses of insulin.

Poverty and Non-Traumatic Amputation

Diabetes is a poor man's disease. Thus, often a diabetes patient has no job, no health insurance, and no family support, and consequently they are severely depressed, and mentally incapacitated. Such persons are destitute for mere living, and understandably, not a living in a healthy lifestyle required for preventing diabetes complications. These are the people who typically develop gangrene of the toes or feet requiring unilateral or bilateral amputation of lower limb. Mortality in these diabetic people is high from incapacitation, recurrent urinary tract infections, and boils and carbuncles. Unilateral or bilateral lower limb amputation is high in the Fiji Islands and Cuba where poverty is prevalent.

In fact, poverty is almost an independent risk factor for diabetic complications exemplified by a high rate of amputation in some segment of population in California, USA, the most resourceful country in the World. Evidence shows that patients residing in low-income households receive lower quality diabetes care, even where Universal coverage for primary health care exists [2].

In the above study done in 2009, one or more non-traumatic amputations was most common in the 45-64 age groups, male, white race, and English speaking people. This study identified 7,973 diabetic lower-extremity amputations in California during the year 2009. Of these 7,205 took place during an inpatient hospitalization and 768 were performed in hospital affiliated outpatient surgery centers. Of this total population, 6,828 (6,094 inpatients and 734 outpatients) experienced one amputation related to diabetes in the study period. Regression analysis of this study shows a strong association between lower-extremity amputation rate and density of low-income households in both Urban and Rural California. Amputation rates varied tenfold between the highest and lowest income neighborhood in the State. I have stated earlier that diabetes is a poor man's disease. To that effect, a recent study showed that poverty and diabetes each contribute independently to vision loss in the United States [3].

Nonetheless, a recent analysis found a reduction in amputation rates per 10,000 people with diabetes in the United States from 58 in 1990 to 28 in 2010 [4]. However, it is apparent that this decrease has not resolved disparities in this debilitating outcome.

Once again, poverty and low income or no income citizens and diabetes complications go hand in hand. The recent expansion of both private insurance and Medicaid enrollment under the affordable care act, address the dimension of access disparity. However, the potential benefits may be blunted by the undersupply of primary care providers in low-income neighborhoods [5].

Renin-Angiotensin Inhibitors Drugs and Dialysis

As stated above due to undersupply of primary care physicians, many Government subsidized Health clinics are run by nurse practitioners. These nurse practitioners as well as primary care physicians have profound gaps in knowledge when it comes to diabetes care. Their knowledge is confined to diagnosis of all adults with Type 2 diabetes and to make out automatic prescriptions of metformin and Lisinopril or glyburide and Lisinopril. Seldom is a prescription of low dose Glargine (Lantus ®) insulin at bedtime offered to some of them. Thus, patients develop all the complications of prolonged uncontrolled hyperglycemia, and on the top of that, use of angiotensin converting enzyme inhibitor (ACEI) and or angiotensin receptor blockers (ARB), resulting in progressive renal failure and dialysis. Here is an example to that effect. A 50-year-old white male was referred to the author from a local Government-sponsored primary care clinic for the finding of low kidney function. He gave history of diabetes for 20 years and a strong family history of diabetes. Indeed a cousin is wheelchair bound and receiving dialysis treatment. His home medications consisted 1) Glargine (Lantus ®) solostar 21 units at night 2.) Aspart insulin (Novolog ®) 7 units with each meal, 3.) Lisinopril 40mg PO daily for 3 years. 4.) Meloxicam-did not take 5.) Other medications with no bearing on diabetes complications. Physical Exam on April 20, 2014 revealed resting pulse 70 beats/min, upright pulse 92 beats/min., sitting blood pressure 140/80 mmHg, upright blood pressure 100/60 mmHg. Laboratory done March 4, 2014 showed Na + 125 mmol/L, K+ 5.3 mmol/L, Fasting Blood Glucose (FBG) 273 mg/dl, serum creatinine (Scr) 1.62 mg/dL with eGFR 49 ml/min, albumin 3.9 g/dL. A repeat testing done on March 6 revealed the following Na+ 122 mmol/L, K + 6.0 mmol/L. FBG 247 mg/dL. Scr 1.59 mg/dL with eGFR 58 ml/min (n=> 60 ml/min). Because of severe postural hypotension, along with severe hyponatremia, hyperkalemia, he was admitted to the hospital for fluid replacement and treatment of hyperkalemia.

Thus, here is a patient who is a victim of a health clinic, which is understaffed with primary care or specialist physicians. Patients may be cared for but inadequately and ineffectively. This type of inadequate and ineffective care is fundamental to development of a variety of acute and chronic diabetes complications. Six weeks following release from the hospital, he had an office visit with the author. His resting pulse was 62 beats/min and sitting and upright blood pressure was 120/80 mmHg. His 2-h postprandial glucose(2hPPG)was 119mg/dL and much improved renal function with serum creatinine decreasing to 1.33 mg/dl and increase of eGFR to normal level 62 ml/min (N= > 60 ml/min). His therapy consisted of Lantus solostar 21 units at bedtime and aspart insulin on a sliding scale. He stopped taking Lisinopril from April 10, 2014, the day he was admitted to hospital. His next office visit with the author was more informative than before, in which severity of diabetes was more clearly defined. The information was presented in Table 1.

Table 1.

July 2014	Fasting	dglucose	2h Postprandial Period
Glucose (mg/dL)	144	203	367
Na + (mmol/L)	138		130
K + (mmol/L)	4.1		4.6
Scr (mg/dL)	1.28		1.41
eGFR (ml/min)	>60		57
UGlucose (0-4+)	2+		4+
U Protein (0-4+)	2+		3+
Serum Magnesium (mg/dL)	1.6		ND
C-peptide (pg/mL)	<0.1		ND

Legend:

U= urine.

Scr= Serum creatinine.

ND = not done.

There is much to learn about diabetes care from Table 1. Glucose levels are elevated with much greater elevation at 2hPPG period (2hPPG-FBG) glucose is elevated. We already reported that dglucose is linked to renal function changes [6]. In this study we showed when dglucose increased by more than 100 mg/dL, d serum creatinine increased between 0.08 and 0.11 mg/dL, and deGFR decreased between 2.73 and 3.73 ml/min when 2hPPG > 200 mg/dL. Thus serum creatinine is 0.13 mg/dL higher in the postprandial period compared to fasting period and eGFR is > 3ml/min lower in the postprandial period compared to fasting. 2+ glucosuria in the fasting period with blood glucose below the glucose threshold (180 mg/dL) indicates a higher milieu of glucose throughout. Severe glycosuria accompanied by greater proteinuria may be interrelated. Hypothetically, reducing hyperglycemia will reduce glycosuria and consequently proteinuria. The very low C-Peptide is a good evidence of insulin deficiency and uncontrolled diabetes, hence requiring higher insulin doses. Finally, discontinuation of Lisinopril allows improvement in renal function, which is evident in this patient.

Among all the complications that emerge from no treatment with insulin or inadequate doses of insulin is renal failure progressing into end stage renal disease (ESRD), which is the costliest to treat, disabling for the patient, and burdensome to family and health care financial providers like Medicare or private insurance companies.

Data from United States ESRD program serves as a testimony to the fact that ACEI/ARB drugs have paved the path to ESRD, requiring dialysis. This is shown in Table 2.

Table 2. Yearly Number of Patients in End Stage Renal Disease (ESRD Program in the United States

Year	**ESRD-Dialysis (Number of patients)**
1978	14,000
1986	32,000
1993	ACEI entered the market
1994	65,000
1998	75,000
ARB entered the market	
2006	354,754
2011	616,000
2020 (Projected)	750,000

ESRD Program = Treatment with Dialysis or Renal Transplantation.

Increasingly more patients are admitted into dialysis clinics. Hence, more profit making private dialysis clinics are opening up in order to accommodate the increasing number of patients with ESRD.

Insulin, a Salutary Treatment of Diabetes for Renal Protection

On the other hand, there are patients who take full responsibility of their illness, hence take insulin as prescribed, and don't develop ESRD or other complications of diabetes as stated before. Here is an example to that effect. A 78-year-old white male consulted the author for diabetes control, so that he can stay healthy and does not have to go to dialysis. He has a long history of diabetes and has been taking Novolin 70/30 55 units before lunch and 40 units before dinner, also takes blood pressure medicine metoprolol 25mg AM and PM, magnesium oxide 400mg PO TID and Niacin 500mg daily.

His laboratory as of May 1, 2014 is shown in Table 3.

Table 3.

	Fasting	**2hPP**
Glucose (mg/dL)	158	177
Scr (mg/dL)	1.50	1.51
eGFR (ml/min)	48	48
BUN (mg/d	22	22
Serum K (mmol/L)	4.7	4.9
Proteinuria	0	0

Dglucose 19 mg/dL

We have shown previously that dglucose less than 100mg/dL with 2hPPG < 200 mg as seen in this patient is associated with insignificant change in renal function. Glucose levels in both periods are higher than normal but the dglucose level determines the renal function changes [6].

Pearl of Wisdom

Though this chapter falls short of many other complications of diabetes but this treatise has presented innovative ideas of glycemic control and prevention of some of the complications of diabetes, such as renal failure requiring the costliest therapy, such as dialysis. This chapter reveals that poverty and non-compliance of the patients and gaps in knowledge of the providers are cumulative factors in the development of diabetic complications. However, a sense of responsibility of the patients themselves for their illness, innovative ideas of the providers, and insulin therapy go a long way to prevent diabetes complications.

References

[1] Gosmanov AR, Gosmanov EO, Dillard-Cannon E. Management of adult diabetic ketoacidosis. Diab Met Syndrome and Obesity: *Targets and Therapt* 2014; 7: 255-264.

[2] Stevens CD, Schriger DL, Raffeto B, Davis AC, Zingmond D, Roby DH. Geographic clustering of diabetic lower-extremity amputations in low-income regions of California *Health Affairs* 2014; 33: 1383-1390.

[3] Ko F, Vitale S, Chou CF, Cotch MF, Saddine J, Friedman DS. Prevalence of non-refractive visual impairment in US adults and associated risk factors. *JAMA* 1999-2002 and 2005-2008. JAMA 2012; 308: 2361-8.

[4] Gregg EW, Li Y, Wang J, Burrows NR, et al. Changes in diabetes-related complications in the United States 1999-2010. *N Engl J Med* 2014; 370: 1514-23.

[5] Bodenheimer T, Pham HH, Primary Care: current problem's and proposed solutions. *Health Aff (Milwood)* 2010; 29: 799-805.

[6] Mandal AK, Hiebert LM, Khamis H, dglucose linked to renal function changes in diabetes. *Diab Res Clin Pract* 2011; 91: 190-194.

Chapter V

Sexual and Urologic Problems of Diabetes

Abstract

Urologic problems and sexual dysfunction are common complications of diabetes mellitus (DM). These complications are in fact a harbinger of the diagnosis of DM. Among elderly men, urinary retention is common, which forces them to seek medical advice when a diagnosis of diabetes is made for the first time. Similarly, overflow urinary incontinence is a common problem encountered in menopausal and elderly women and is often attributed to bladder prolapse due to weakness of pelvic muscles in multiparous women. This may be the case but it seems to be more prevalent in those women who also have DM. Sexual dysfunction is equally common in men and women with DM. However, sexual dysfunction in terms of erectile dysfunction (ED) is detected more frequently in men than women. This is due to the social stigma for women not to discuss sexual dysfunction with their doctors. Equally important is the fact that medical professionals seldom ask questions about sexual activity during history and physical examination.

Urologic problems, if not detected, could add to renal function deterioration, which is common in DM. On the other hand, sexual dysfunction does not have a direct impact on the organ function but it affects the psychosocial aspect of the family. Therefore, diabetes care involves total care of the patient including post care. Kidney function and cardiac assessment as ED is known to precede coronary artery disease. Similarly, in all cases of urinary retention, urinary incontinence and urinary tract infection, DM should always be considered as the underlying cause and testing should be done to rule out DM.

Introduction

Urinary frequency, difficulty in urination or inability to pass urine (urinary retention) and changes in sexual function are common health problems with the aging process. Having diabetes can mean early onset and increased severity of these problems. Urologic and sexual complications of diabetes occur because of the damage diabetes can cause to the blood vessels and nerves. Men with diabetes have difficulty with erection or ejaculation. Women with diabetes have difficulty with sexual response to partner, and vaginal lubrication. People who can keep their diabetes under control with diet and insulin can minimize their urinary and sexual complications.

Diabetes and Urologic Complications

More than half of men and women with diabetes have bladder dysfunction because of nerve damage that controls bladder function. Bladder dysfunction can have a profound effect on a person's quality of life. Common bladder problems in men and women with diabetes include the following.

a) *Urine retention:* Urinary retention is a very common problem in undiagnosed diabetes or diabetes treated with oral antidiabetic agents. Nerve damage keeps the bladder muscles from not getting the message that is time to urinate or makes the muscles too weak to empty the bladder. Urinary retention may also lead to overflow incontinence or leakage of urine when the bladder is full and does not empty properly. Incomplete emptying of the bladder leads to back up of the urine to the ureters and the renal pelvis eventually leading to dilation of the kidney called hydronephrosis and renal failure.
b) Bladder dysfunction

   Danesgari et al. [1] presented the "temporal theory of diabetic bladder dysfunction", which proposes that hyperglycemia-induced polyuria plays a major pathophysiologic role during the early stages of diabetes polyuria, causing compensatory bladder hypertrophy and associated myogenic and neurogenic alterations with time and accumulation of toxic metabolites, decompensation of bladder tissue and function ensues, resulting in the classical signs and symptoms of diabetic cystopathy (hypocontractile detrusor or atonic bladder) in patients with urinary voiding problems.

A study by Lee et al. [2] compared the voiding behavior of 194 women with diabetes compared with 162 control women using a lower urinary tract symptoms questionnaire and uroflowmetry. They found that diabetic women had significantly higher nocturia scores, weaker urinary streams, reduced voided volumes and lower maximal flow rates.

Diabetes has been identified as an independent risk factor for urinary incontinence that leads to significant distress and poorer quality of life.

An epidemiological study suggests that diabetes independently increases the risk of urinary incontinence in women, and it is 50% to 200% more common in women with diabetes than in women with normal glucose levels.

a) *Poor control of sphincter muscles:* sphincter muscles surround the urethra and keep it closed to hold urine in the bladder. If the nerves to the sphincter muscles are damaged, the muscles may weaken causing incontinence of urine or may tighten the sphincter causing retention of urine. It is important to understand that incomplete emptying of the bladder may lead to recurrent attacks of infection in the bladder (cystitis) and or in the kidneys (pyelonephritis)

Diabetes Related Urinary Tract Infection

Urinary tract infection universally described as UTI is due to bacteria migrating from the digestive tract to the Urinary tract. UTI is more common in females due to the proximity of the urethral opening to the anal opening. UTI may occur in the form of urethritis, cystitis, or pyelonephritis. Symptoms of UTI include

- A frequent urge to urinate
- Pain or burning in the bladder or urethra during urination (dysuria)
- Cloudy or reddish urine
- In women pressure above the pubic bone
- In men, a feeling of fullness in the rectum.

Frequent urination is due to 3+ to 4+ glucose in urine in untreated or uncontrolled diabetes. This must be distinguished from painful urination due to UTI. Unlike urethritis or cystitis, pyelonephritis gives rise to fever with chills, pain in the back or side and nausea and vomiting.

A scientific study from India [3] determined the clinical features, microbiological profiles, prognostic factors, and treatment outcome of pyelonephritis in 105 patients with diabetes. Patients were treated with appropriate antibiotics and percutaneous drainage as required. This study described both emphysematous pyelonephritis (EPN) and non-EPN (NEPN). In this population, 75.2% had NEPN and 24.7% EPN. Escherichia Coli (E. Coli) was most common organism. Those with EPN had a higher incidence of uncontrolled diabetes and were resistant to antibiotic therapy alone requiring percutaneous drainage more often. Patients with EPN had a poorer treatment outcome compared to those with NEPN. However, the mortality was not different between the two groups [3].

Diabetes and Sexual Dysfunction

a) Sexual dysfunction in men with Diabetes
b) Sexual dysfunction in women with Diabetes

A. Sexual Dysfunction in Men

Sexual dysfunction in men is connoted as erectile dysfunction or ED. ED is the consistent inability to have an erection firm enough for satisfactory sexual intercourse. The condition includes the total inability to have an erection and the inability to sustain an erection. Estimates of the prevalence of ED in men with diabetes varies widely ranging from 20 to 75 percent. Men who have diabetes are two or three times more likely to have ED than men who do not have diabetes. Among men with ED, those with diabetes may experience the problem as much as to 10 to 15 years earlier than men without diabetes. Research suggests that ED may be an early marker of diabetes, particularly in men ages 45 and younger.

As noted by Ficher [4], the first documentation of impotence and diabetes was made by Rollo in 1798. In 1906, Naunyn noted impotence to be the most common symptom in diabetic men.

McCulloch et al. [5] reported that 9 percent of 88 diabetic men ages 20 to 29 complained of impotence. By age 70 and older, impotence was noted in more than 95 percent of diabetic men (unpublished observations). ED does not appear to be related to the duration of diabetes and may precede the occurrence of other complications. Once ED develops, it seems to be permanent.

B. Sexual Dysfunction in Women with Diabetes

Women with diabetes experience sexual dysfunction as much as men but it is unreported. Women feel ashamed to talk about their low sexual desire or poor sexual performance with their doctors. On the other hand, doctors seldom ask categorically about the sexual function in their patients, men or women. Thus, the pattern of sexual dysfunction in women with diabetes is thinly documented.

Sexual dysfunction in women may include:

- Decreased vaginal lubrication
- Uncomfortable or painful sexual intercourse
- Decreased or no desire for sexual activity
- Decreased or absent sexual response.

Decreased or absent sexual response includes the inability to become or remain aroused, reduced or no sensation in the genital area, and the inability to reach orgasm.

Causes of sexual dysfunction in women with diabetes include nerve damage, reduced blood flow to genital and vaginal tissues, and hormonal changes. Other possible causes are antihypertensive drugs, alcohol abuse, smoking, psychological problems such as anxiety or depression, gynecologic infections and conditions related to pregnancy or menopause.

The mechanism of ED is somewhat elusive. However, the most convincing evidence is the association between glycemic control and ED. To that effect, this particular study is helpful for direct patient care. This study was undertaken at the Cleveland Veterans Affairs Medical Center. Patients completed questions 1 to 5 of the International Index of Erectile Function. The primary outcome measure was erectile function score. The mean subject age was 62 ± 12.3 years, the mean HbA1c was 8.1 ± 1.9%, and the mean ED score was 16.6 ± 5.9 (range to 5 to 23). Stratified analysis revealed that the mean ED score decreased as HbA1c increased (0.002). The test for linearity was also significant (P=0.001). Multivariate analysis showed that HbA1c was an independent predictor of ED even after adjusting for peripheral neuropathy. Finally, this study asserted that ED correlates with the level of glycemic control. Peripheral neuropathy and HbA1c but not patients' age were independent predictors of erectile dysfunction [6].

Risk Factors for Developing Sexual and Urologic Problems of Diabetes

Risk factors are conditions that increase the chances of getting a particular disease. The more risk factors people have, the greater their chances of developing the disease or condition. Diabetes related sexual and urologic problems appear to be more common in people who:

- Have poor blood glucose control
- Have high levels of blood cholesterol
- Have high blood pressure
- Are overweight
- Are older than 40 years
- Smoker
- Are physically inactive

Sexual Dysfunction in Diabetes: A Taboo Not Limited to Men

Nearly half of all men and women living with diabetes experience some sort of sexual dysfunction. Many studies have evidenced the negative impact of diabetes on normal sexual functioning especially on the quality of life among men who indicate sexual dysfunction as a main complication. In rural Uganda, men are often heard saying, "I am no longer a man" (due to lack of sexual function) to describe how diabetes informs their self-perception. Therefore, the lack of attention to diabetes related sexual dysfunction cannot be ascribed to either the magnitude of or the perceptions about the importance of the complication. Culturally, discussing sexual dysfunction is often taboo and people with diabetes can be very reluctant to share their sexual problems. A study found that only 19% of women and 47% of men experiencing sexual dysfunction related to diabetes have discussed the issue with a physician. When people with diabetes are exposed to the facts about the nature and prevalence of diabetes-related sexual dysfunction, they find ways to overcome the taboo and seek solutions to the problem. Therefore, more research and open communication of the finding could increase awareness of sexual dysfunction among practitioners and people living with diabetes [7].

Pathophysiology and Mechanism of ED: Association with Coronary Syndrome

Presence of hypertension, cardiovascular disorder, and peripheral neuropathy increase the risk of ED. With the recognition that endothelial dysfunction is the common denominator linking vascular disease to ED came the realization that ED may not just be a consequence of vascular disease, especially coronary disease – a sentinel. The smaller penile arteries (1-2 mm diameter) potentially suffer from plaque burden and/or endothelial dysfunction symptomatically earlier than larger coronary artery (3-4mm), carotid (5-7mm) and ileofemoral (6-8 mm) arteries, as a consequence ED may act as a marker for silent coronary artery disease and therefore precede a coronary event. ED could be a predictor of an acute event as well as being the manifestation of more advanced chronic diseases. This concept is reinforced by ED and vascular disease, which share the same risk factors: diabetes, smoking, hypertension, hyperlipidemia, obesity, depression and lack of physical activity [8].

It is has been noted that multivessel CAD, and chronic coronary syndrome are independent predictors of ED and in those with acute presentation, the prevalence of ED was linked to the extent of CAD-again ED coming before the CAD presentation in the majority by 2-3 years.

The second Princeton consensus conference focused on sexual dysfunction and cardiac risk and concluded that ED is a warning sign of vascular disease with the practical recommendation that a man with ED and no cardiac symptoms is a cardiac or vascular patient until proved otherwise [9].

Endothelial Dysfunction

The endothelium is vital to the maintenance of vascular health. Nitric Oxide (NO) is the most potent vasodilator and is secreted by the endothelium. It is synthesized from L-arginine by the endothelial enzyme NO synthase. NO released in response to sexual stimulation relaxes the penile vascular smooth muscle by increasing the intracellular cyclic 3’, 5’ guanosine monophosphate (CGMP) concentration. Vasodilatation of the erectile tissues allows the sinusoidal spaces to fill with blood resulting in the attainment and maintenance of an erection. The presence of peripheral neuropathy also increases the risk of ED, possibly because of undiagnosed autonomic neuropathy: almost 100% of patients with diabetic autonomic neuropathy will have ED. The interaction between endothelial dysfunction and autonomic neuropathy results in an inability to increase blood flow under conditions of stress or increased demands, such as during an erection [10].

Prevention and Treatment of Sexual and Urologic Problems in Diabetes

A. *Non-pharmacologic Intervention.* Being physically active and maintaining a healthy weight can also prevent the long-term complications of diabetes. For those who smoke, quitting will lower the risk of developing sexual and urologic problems due to nerve damage and also lower the risk for other health problems related to diabetes, including CAD, stroke and kidney disease.

Erectile dysfunction can be managed in a diabetes clinic or general practice surgery. Few investigations are required: Fasting and 2hPP basic metabolic panel (BMP), glycosylated hemoglobin, serum testosterone and prolactin level. BMP provides glucose levels to determine the severity of diabetes and state of renal function and electrolyte pattern. Serum testosterone levels determine if hypogonadism co-exists with diabetes. Restoring potency to try and save a failing relationship is seldom successful and makes matters worse. Psychosexual counseling is advised in failing relationships as well as in cases involving depression, severe anxiety, loss of attraction between partners, fears of intimacy or performance anxiety. Spontaneous reversal of erectile dysfunction in diabetes is rare, so treatment is long-term. Changing medication to improve erectile function is usually not worthwhile in men with diabetes, unless, there is a strong temporal relationship between the start of treatment and the onset of the problem.

There is a growing evidence of a link between late-onset male hypogonadism and diabetes and the metabolic syndrome. The prevalence of hypogonadism is increased in diabetes. Thus, testosterone replacement improves erectile function and response to phosphodiesterase type 5 (PDE5) inhibitor in hypogonadal men [11].

Lifestyle Changes and Exercise

Lifestyle changes have been shown to improve endothelial function to improve in patients with diabetes. Epidemiological studies have identified sedentary lifestyle as a potential modifiable risk factor in men with ED and provide moderate support for the beneficial role of increasing exercise [10].

Pharmacologic Intervention

Although spontaneous return of sexual function in patients with diabetes with ED is rare, attempts must be made to treat diabetes with insulin therapy.

As a first step diagnosis of diabetes with 2hPP, BMP must be made. Patients with a random diagnosis of diabetes may not have established diabetes. 2hPPG > 200mg/dL establishes the diagnosis of diabetes. BMP provides information if kidney function is normal or abnormal. Abnormal renal function increases the risk of ED. Although evidence is lacking that intensive insulin therapy will reverse ED, our cell culture investigation in diabetes is a testimony to the repair of vascular damage with insulin therapy in diabetes. Therefore, it is important that we treat established diabetes with intensive insulin therapy with a hope to regain sexual function by keeping 2hPPG < 200mg/dL or with d (delta) of less than 100 mg/dL [12].

It is evident from personal observation by intensive care of patients with diabetes that urinary retention and urinary incontinence improve significantly by treating diabetes with intensive insulin therapy. Actually, decreasing glucosuria by controlling hyperglycemia with insulin therapy will decrease polyuria, nocturia, urinary retention, and urinary incontinence. As of now, there is no evidence to indicate that the treatment of diabetes with oral antidiabetic agents will improve urinary symptoms. The reason for that is that oral antidiabetic agents do not lower 2hPPG [13].

For other pharmacologic interventions including PDE-5 inhibitors, intravencavernosal therapy, intraurethral prostaglandin therapy, surgery, the author refers the patients to a Urologist.

Author is convinced that intensive therapy in diabetes will restore sexual function but therapy in diabetes will last for a long time.

Another interesting point to make is that patients with ED must have a full cardiovascular assessment and in case of documented CAD, increasing coronary blood flow by stenting or bypass surgery could improve sexual function. A clinical trial to that effect may unravel the association.

Pearl of Wisdom

Sexual dysfunction and urologic problems such as urinary retention and urinary incontinence are common accompaniments of uncontrolled diabetes. Control of diabetes with insulin improves urinary problems but does not necessarily restore sexual function. Nevertheless, it is important to know that insulin is the mainstay of therapy for these disorders.

References

[1] Daneshgaru F, LivG, Birder L, Hanna-Mitchell AT, Chacko S. Diabetic bladder dysfunction current translational knowledge. *J Urol* 2009; 182: S18-26/

[2] Lee WC, WO HP, Tai Ty Liv SP, Chin J, Yu HF. Effects of diabetes on female voiding behavior *J Urol* 2004; 172: 989-92

[3] Kumar S, Ramaclandran R, Mete U, et al. Acute pyelonephritis in diabetes mellitus: single center experience. *Indian J Nephrol* 2014; 24: 367-371

[4] Ficher M, Zuckerman M, Fishkin RE et al. Do endocrines play an etiologic role in diabetic and nondiabetic sexual dysfunction? *J Androl* 1984; 5: 8-16

[5] Mcculloch DK, Campbell W, WUFC et al. The prevalence of diabetic impotence. *Diabetologia* 1980; 18: 279-283.

[6] Romeo JH, Seftel Ad, Madhun ZT, Aron DC. Sexual dysfunction in men with diabetes Type 2: Association with glycemic control. *J Urol* 2000; 163: 788-791

[7] Nielsen J, Nielsen KK. Letter to Editor. Diab Res Clin Pract 2014: 103:

[8] Jackson G. Erectile dysfunction: a marker of silent coronary disease EU *Heart J:* 2006; 27:2613-2614.

[9] Matorsi P, Ravagni PM, Gallis et al. Association between Erectile dysfunction and coronary artery disease. Role of coronary clinical presentation and extent of coronary vessels involvement: The COBRA trial. *Eur Heart J* 2006; 27: 2632-2639.

[10] Thethi TK, Asafu-Adjaye No, Fonseca VA. *Erectile dysfunction Clin* Diabetes 2005; 23: 105-113.

[11] Price D, Sexual problems in diabetes. *Medicine* 2014; 43: 38-40.

[12] Mandal AK, Hiebert LM, Khamis H. dglucose relates to renal function changes in diabetes Diabetes. *Diab Res Clin Pract* 2011; 91: 190-194.

[13] Effect of Metformin compared to Insulin in renal preservation of adults with diabetes presented in American Society of Nephrology. November 15, 2015, Philadephia.

Chapter VI

Too Many Controversies Seriously Affecting Salutary Diabetes Care

Abstract

Prevention of the complications of diabetes is needed because complications are disabling, and the enormous cost of treating diabetic complications is imposing a serious economic burden on the health care system throughout the world. The rate of complications, for example, end stage renal disease – related to diabetes is escalating mainly due to controversies affecting diagnosis and therapy of diabetes. In most cases, diagnosis of diabetes is not confirmed by 2h postprandial glucose (2hPPG) and then treatment using oral anti-diabetics agents as the prevalent therapy. Over time exhaustion of pancreatic beta cells ensue and the result is overt diabetes accompanied by one or more complications such as foot ulcer or heart attack. The underlying factors for the adversary in diabetes care are profound gaps of knowledge in understanding the pathobiology of diabetes among the professionals and the high influence of commercialism in the clinical practice of diabetes. It is important to overturn the commercial bias and order 2hPPG using the basic metabolic panel, which will also provide renal function parameters. Diagnosis of diabetes must be affirmed by 2hPPG $\geq$ 200mg/dL ($\geq$ 11.1mmol/L) and treating patients with confirmed diabetes by insulin therapy, which will invariably prevent most or all of the complications of diabetes.

Introduction

Diabetes mellitus (DM) or diabetes as the common term is the biggest challenge in current clinical practice. Challenge means the utmost attention is required by the professionals as the most important task in diabetes care, which is prevention of complications of diabetes, namely blindness; amputation of toes or a limb; kidney failure and dialysis; heart attack; and sexual dysfunction. A cure for diabetes, as is commonly talked about, is far-fetched, but prevention of the complications is attainable.

Prevention of the complications is needed because they are disabling, and the enormous cost of treating diabetes complications is imposing a severe economic burden on health care systems throughout the world. Diabetes, like high blood pressure, is a silent disease – in particular, in adults – and the damage caused to the organs by high glucose is an insidious process. Thus, the damage remains undetected for a long time, but manifests severely in the late stage. The damage caused by high glucose to the organs is fairly uniform both in children, young adults, and in older adults and the elderly. However, symptoms can be explosive in children and young adults due to polyuria, polydipsia, and rapid loss of weight. On the other hand, manifestations can be subtle in adults. Adults often do not know they have diabetes until symptoms manifest due to the damage to an organ. Some of the symptoms, not in any order, are urinary retention, sexual dysfunction, decreased vision, chest pain, protein in urine or decreased kidney function found on routine physical examination, recurrent urinary tract infection, non-healing foot ulcers or discoloration of a foot or toes. In fact, diabetes is often detected for the first time in patients brought into the emergency of a hospital for chest pain and found to have acute coronary syndrome.

1. Controversies Affecting Care

There are controversies concerning diabetic nephropathy versus other complications of diabetes. Numerous studies in the past have confirmed that tight glycemic control with multiple insulin injections prevent microvascular and macrovascular complications of diabetes (1-4). Since glucose bathes the entire vascular system involving all organs, the injury is likely to be uniform in all organs. Our cell culture studies using normal glucose of 90 mg/dL (5mmol/L) and high glucose of 540mg/dL (30mmol/L) for treatment of vascular endothelial cells show no damage or severe damage, respectively (5). Our cell culture studies also revealed that the addition of insulin, along with a high concentration of glucose, abrogated the damage.

Thus, we have developed a hypothesis:

Damaged endothelial cells shed off into capillary Lumina

⇩

calcification of necrotic tissue with occlusion of capillary lumina

⇩

Ischemia of the organ

This is a slow ischemia, giving rise to fibrotic changes in the heart, kidneys, and peripheral vessels. In the kidney glomerular sclerosis and interstitial fibrosis gives rise to chronic renal failure and end stage renal disease (ESRD). Here is a patient illustrated to that effect. A 58-year-old African American male was admitted into a local hospital in early December 2014 with vague symptoms. He was found to have developed acute renal failure (ARF). He gave history of hypertension and 14 years history of diabetes. He was treated with Glucotrol (glyburide) 5mg daily for diabetes and amlodipine 5mg daily for hypertension. At the time of hospital admission, his serum creatinine was 5mg/dL and CPK was mildly elevated. Thus, rhabdomyolysis was considered as the cause of renal failure. He received normal saline infusion and atenolol 50mg PO daily and clonidine 0.1mg PO TID for blood pressure control. During the hospital course his serum creatinine increased further to 5.9mg/dL with eGFR of 11ml/min. Serum electrolytes were normal. His hemoglobin rapidly decreased to 7.9g/dL requiring packed cell transfusion. Serum glucose levels (fasting) in the hospital were normal 111mg/dL and 98mg/dL. Thus, rapidly progressive glomerulonephritis was considered. A 24-hour urinary protein was 2.4g. A kidney biopsy was performed and studied by light and immunofluorescence microscopy. Light microscopy showed 13 glomeruli to be globally sclerotic out of 31 glomeruli. Well-established nodular expansion of merangial matrix is noted; capillary loop basement membrane is thickened. No deposit or necrosis was noted.

There is severe interstitial fibrosis with associated tubular atrophy, involving over half the cortical surface area. Diffuse lymphocytic infiltrate was identified throughout the interstitium. Focally severe hyaline sclerosis of arterioles is noted. On immunofluorescence, kappa and lambda light chains were negative.

Here is a representative light microscopy picture of the kidney biopsy, showing typical nodular glomerulosclerosis and severe tubular atrophy and interstitial changes (PAS stain).

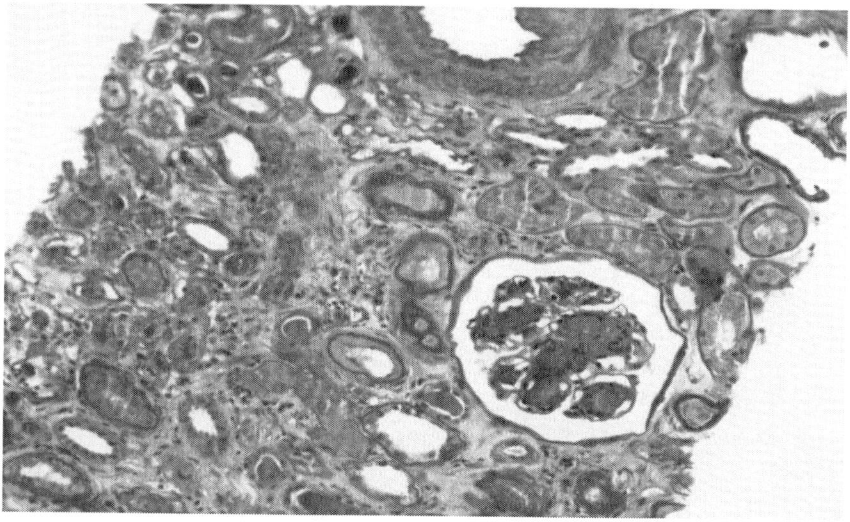

An office visit 5 days after hospital discharge showed slight edema and elevated blood pressure 170/100 mmHg. His renal function is slightly improved serum creatinine 4.60mg/dL with eGFR of 14ml/min. Serum albumin is 2.7g/dL. He feels fine. His current therapy consists of atenolol 50mg PO daily, omeprazole 20mg PO daily, clonidine 0.1mg PO TID and Bumex 2mg PO twice daily. He will return to the office in three weeks.

Here is a great example of controversies affecting diabetes care. If he was treated with insulin and hypertension was better controlled, he may not have developed advanced diabetic nephropathy associated with end stage renal failure.

In the heart, coronary artery occlusion gives rise to angina. In the extremities, foot ulcer and gangrene supervene. In the retina microaneurysm is formed. Therefore, our cell culture studies have prompted us to develop a unified theory, which is similar to other authors (6). Therefore, if we can agree with the unified theory, our focus will be directed to control of hyperglycemia to reduce the risk of complications. It is intriguing to think why glucose at a high level – for instance≥ 200mg/dL (≥11.1mmol/L) causes damage to the organs, whereas similar glucose at a normal level does not. Therefore an important question can be asked: if glucose in and of itself has any direct effect in causing tissue damage or whether a high level of glucose does so by altering cellular oxygenation. Thus, a plausible mechanism of cellular injury is inhibition of the glutathione pathway by high glucose environment. An excessive number of oxygen-free radicals produced by reduced glutathione could play an important role in widespread organ damage in diabetes (7). In our laboratory, cultured endothelial cells were treated with inhibitor of glutathione, buthioninesulfoxamine, which showed endothelial cell damage similar to that induced by high glucose (8), thereby supporting the glutathione inhibition theory in the pathogenesis of glucose-induced endothelial cell damage.

Although the exact mechanism with regard to organ damage caused by high glucose is yet to be unraveled, as of now, we know for sure that sustained elevation of blood glucose level ≥200mg/dL (≥11.1mmol/L) unequivocally causes organ damage producing the gamut of complications already stated.

2. Distortion in the Paradigm of Diabetes Therapy

There are several important factors underlying distortion in effective glycemic control hence culminating in development of serious complications

These factors are:

- Gaps in knowledge
- Prevalent use of HbA1c in the assessment of glycemic control
- No attention to outcome measures
- Preponderant use of oral anti-diabetic agents in treatment of diabetes

There are profound gaps of knowledge in the treatment of diabetes. In the diagnosis and management of diabetes fasting blood glucose and HbA1c are most commonly ordered. Importance of 2h postprandial glucose (2hPPG) in management of diabetes is seldom acknowledged. Thus, 2hPPG is unknown to most professionals.

Author's Studies Comprise Mostly 2hPPG

Most professionals order quarterly HbA1c. In author's studies, HbA1c correlates well with 2hPPG but glucosylated hemoglobin is subject to variations with hemoglobin levels. Thus, anemic persons will reveal low HbA1c levels even though they may be overtly diabetic. Hemoglobin levels are frequently low in diabetes with chronic kidney disease although their diabetes control is poor. Considering all these pitfalls, 2hPPG is a pivotal test for treating diabetes and monitoring glycemic control.

Outcome measures are limited to cardiovascular disorders consisting of myocardial infarction or death associated with 2hPPG ≥200mg/dL (9). Even the DECODE study showed that risk of cardiovascular death increases threefold as 2-h post challenge glucose levels increase from 54mg/dL to 199mg/dL, although these readings are in the non-diabetic range. Once again, 2-h post challenge glucose levels are determinant of cardiovascular outcomes and possibly other outcomes, which were not tested. Few investigators, including the author himself, tested the relationship between 2-h PPG and renal function changes. A single study from Italy found that 2hPPG greater than 200mg/dL (11.1 mmol/L) and HbA1c above 8% (established diabetes) is closely linked to rapid decrease in GFR; whereas a 2hPPG of less than 200mg/dL and HbA1c of less than 8% is associated with trivial or no change in GFR (10). Our data is consistent with the report from Italy. In addition we innovated d(delta) glucose (2hPPG-PBG), which is a stronger predicator of renal function changes than 2-hPPG. We have shown that dglucose above 100mg/dL is associated with significant increase of serum creatinine. Most importantly, we did not find any correlation between HbA1c and renal function changes [11]. In other words, it is a mistake to use HbA1c as a marker of glycemic control when following diabetes patients who have developed renal failure. Other studies have shown that reduced 2hPPG is strongly associated with reduction in retinopathy and nephropathy [12].

Despite the great importance of 2hPPG asserted in the outcome measures of cardiovascular disorders, albeit with some progress in the assessment of renal failure, HbA1c continues to be the standard test for evaluation of diabetes control. An apparent reason for this solidarity is a commercial bias because most oral anti-diabetic agents reduce HbA1c but not 2PPG. We have unpublished data to that effect. Oral anti-diabetic agents are the target therapy for diabetes prescribed by general practitioners, internists and endocrinologists or diabetologists. In that regard, it is important to know that the American Association of Clinical Endocrinologists/American College of Endocrinology consensus panel on type 2 diabetes mellitus asserted that in order to minimize the risk of diabetes-related complications, the goal of therapy is to achieve an HbA1c of 6.5% or less. This panel considered monotherapy, dual therapy, and triple therapy with oral anti-diabetic agents and with insulin as the last item in the list [13]. As soon as the diagnosis of diabetes is made in the office or clinic, the typical sequence of events is a prescription of metformin 500mg twice daily increasing to 1000mg twice daily if HbA1c is not 6.5% or less. Thereafter glyburide 10mg twice daily or pioglitazone 15-30mg twice daily is added to the regimen to promote glycemic control. With the introduction of incretin therapy, a DPP-4 inhibitor is added when the glucose levels are still elevated despite dual or triple therapy and the patients already had developed complications, which are already stated. Then they are advised to consider taking insulin in an inadequate dose such as a nightly dose of 15-20 units Glargine insulin (Lantus). An important question is why insulin is advised so late in the process. A low dose of insulin and late in the process is unlikely to reverse the complication or repair the damage done. Here again comes the commercial bias deterring the doctors to prescribe insulin.

3. Major Distortion and the Worst Controversy in Therapy of Diabetes

A major distortion and the worst controversy lay in the management of diabetic nephropathy and renal failure. Diabetic nephropathy is manifested by no to heavy proteinuria, depending on the duration of diabetes, adequacy of glycemic control and therapy used to achieve glycemic controls. In general, the longer the duration of uncontrolled or untreated diabetes, in particular with reference to glycemic level consistently above 200mg/dL (≥11.1mmol/L), and no insulin rejuvenation, the more likely heavy proteinuria will be found. In authors studies, insulin treated diabetic patients reveal no proteinuria or 1+ proteinuria. Uncommonly few show 2+ proteinuria. This mild proteinuria has no impact on renal function in the author's patients. Other authors reported that mild proteinuria or quantitatively less than 500mg 24-hour proteinuria has no adverse effect on renal function [14].

However, a previous study swung the pendulum from glycemic control to minimal proteinuria (microalbuminuria) control in diabetes. This rat study showed that hyperglycemia causes hyperfiltration, and hyperfiltration is associated with microalbuminuria and glomerulosclerosis. They hypothesized that by reducing microalbuminuria with angiotensin converting enzyme inhibitors (ACEI), glomerulosclerosis or diabetic nephropathy will be mitigated (15). Thereafter a clinical study was done in which diabetes patients were treated with the ACEI captopril and found doubling of serum creatinine in fewer captopril treated versus the control group. The HbA1C levels were above 11% in both groups. 2hPPG levels were not provided and whether these patients were treated with insulin was not stated. Thus, by showing fewer captopril treated patients developing ESRD (End Stage Renal Disease) this study revolutionized microalbuminuria as a standard test for diabetes and therapy with ACEI drugs as a standard of care for diabetes [16].

In the current day practice, glucose control, which is fundamental to prevention strategies, has taken the back seat; whereas, ACEI and angiotensin receptor blocker (ARB) drugs have taken the forefront in the marketplace. Given the widespread consensus of ACEI/ARB as renoprotective drugs, insulin rejuvenation is considered an old fashioned therapy. This trapped position of glucose control combined with the deceptive consensus of ACEI/ARB as a frontier therapy of diabetes – has resulted in increased incidence of ESRD and opening of growing numbers of private dialysis clinics to treat the ESRD patients. All these are lucrative for the professionals and the industry, but tragic for the patients and their families.

Most patients who develop ESRD are automatically started on dialysis therapy, even though they are asymptomatic and exhibit no fluid, electrolytes or acid-based disorders. Maintenance dialysis therapy prolongs survival, but this survival is less than optimal and associated with more time in hospitals than at home (17), and the expenditures from taxpayer financed programs and personal insurance are far out of proportion to the quality of survival. For instance, dialysis therapy in the USA is exhausting Medicare and Medicaid budgets, leaving fewer dollars for prevention strategies. Further, the progressive physical burden and mental anguish imposed on the loved ones and the demands of in-home care associated with pre- and post-dialysis treatments are detrimental to the family. Combining all of these adverse outcomes, a serious question can be raised about the overall benefit of chronic dialysis therapy in diabetes.

On the other hand, ESRD is largely preventable with adequate control of hyperglycemia (glucose level of < 200mg/dL or < 11.1mmol/L) by intensive insulin therapy implemented early in the course of diabetes and the control of hypertension by antihypertensive therapy without the use of ACEI/ARB drugs. It is needless to underscore that ACEI/ARB drugs are not renoprotective [18].

4. Therapy by Oral Anti-diabetic Agents

Oral anti-diabetic agents are good in lowering fasting glucose but practically ineffective in lowering the postprandial glucose surge. At least, no evidence exists to that effect. Postprandial glucose surge does not necessarily cause any unusual symptoms immediately, thus not alerting the patients or the professionals to take any action. However, patients who home monitor their glucose levels regularly find out that their glucose is not under control with oral anti-diabetic drugs, which leads to emergency room visits, or consultations with another doctor to get advice for a different, albeit better treatment, for good glucose control.

Since postprandial glycemic surge does not produce symptoms and if patients refuse to take insulin because of fear of injections, professionals and pharmaceutical companies are at an advantageous position to exploit the ignorance of the patients with regard to the seriousness of uncontrolled hyperglycemia. Hence, it has become a standard practice to prescribe multiple oral anti-diabetic agents to keep HbA1C at 6.5% or less [13] thereby making the patients happy with a false sense of security, while returning again and again to their doctors' office. Preaching treatment with insulin again and again carries a distinct risk for the doctors of losing the patients, and hence the income.

What can we do to overturn the current practice of diabetes care and treat patients appropriately to ensure a successful journey to control diabetes and not crash somewhere in the middle of the trip, as is happening now with amputation, ESRD or heart attack? Here is one idea to that effect: Patients who have understood that good glucose control with insulin is permissive of a healthy life can be considered a significant part of prevention strategies. Therefore, prevention strategies comprise:

1. Group therapy through volunteerism of insulin-treated patients who are doing well with other patients who have refused home monitoring of glucose who should take insulin injections. It will be an innovative step in order to increase the number of patients who take insulin and keep glucose under control. It is like a clinical trial, except diabetic patients who are taking insulin will act as counselors to the patients who have refused to take insulin, to make them understand how uncontrolled diabetes can jeopardize their life and how well-controlled diabetes with insulin therapy can permit them to live a

healthy life. The volunteerism is attainable and will be the least expensive, albeit the most profitable, part of diabetes care. This approach is also likely to reduce the rate of intentional insulin omission [19].

2. Adequate glucose control by prescribed insulin therapy consisting of insulin Glargine or detemir after breakfast and dinner, and regular insulin before each meal to reduce post-meal excursions [20].
3. Adequate control of hypertension by antihypertensive drug therapy singly or in combination, for example, beta blocker, calcium channel blocker and vasodilators. They are safe and effective;
4. Avoidance of ACEI/ARB drugs. It is fundamentally wrong to prescribe these drugs as renoprotective drugs and ignore glucose control, which is critical in prevention strategy;
5. Shift focus away from microalbuminuria control and give full attention to total care of the diabetic patient with details to bladder function, foot care, sexual function, cardiovascular health, cognitive function and finally overall quality of life;
6. Frequent office visits are an integral part of total diabetes care, as stated above. Diabetes patients often have the illusion of going into dialysis. Professionals must counsel the patients to invalidate such illusion. Dialysis should be considered as an accident and not a part of routine diabetes therapy.

Conclusion

It is evident from the preponderance of literature that more attention is paid to HbA1C levels than to any other glycemic parameter related to diabetes control. This is regrettable as our own studies and many others have shown that when 2-hour postprandial glucose is used as the leading measurement for glycemic control in conjunction with insulin injection over oral anti-diabetic agents, the outcome measurements are greatly improved. Renal function in particular remains stable and in many cases, is improved (20). Cardiovascular disorders may also be forestalled with the use of insulin therapy over oral anti-diabetic drugs [21].

Perhaps the most important point to make in this commentary is that the physicians and the patients must work hand in hand. It is the physician's responsibility to encourage insulin therapy either when diabetes is first diagnosed or promptly when oral therapy fails, thereby avoiding beta cell exhaustion and death. This will ensure stability of metabolic control and reduce complications related to metabolic abnormalities, which will translate into improved overall health, improved quality of life with decreased comorbidities, and a longer life expectancy [22].

References

[1] Reichard P., Berglund B., Britz, A., Cars I., Nilsson B.Y., Rosenqvist U., Intensified conventional insulin treatment tetrads the microvascular complications of IDDIABETES (insulin-dependent diabetes mellitus): The SDIS (Stockholm Diabetes Intervention Study) after 5 years, *J Intern Med.*1991; 230: 101-108.

[2] Soper C.P, Barron J.L., Hyer S.L., Long-term glycemic control directly correlates with glomerular filtration rate in early type 1 diabetes mellitus before the onset of microalbuminuria, *Diabet. Med.*1998 15 : 1010-1014.

[3] Fabre J., Balant L.P., Dayer P.G., Fox H.M., Vernet A.T., The kidney in maturity onset diabetes mellitus: A clinical study of 510 patients, *Kidney Int.* 1982; 21:730-738.

[4] The Diabetes Control and Complications Trial Research Group, The effect of intensive treatment of diabetes on the development and progression of long-term complications in insulin-dependent diabetes mellitus, *N. Engl. J. Med.* 1993;329:977-980.

[5] Mandal A.K., Puchalski J.T., Lemley-Gillespie S., Taylor C.A., Kohna M., Effect of insulin and heparin on glucose-induced vascular damage in cell culture, *Kidney Int.* 200;57: 2492-2501.

[6] Brownlee M., Pathobiology of diabetic complications: A unifying mechanism, *Diabetes* 2005; 54:1615-1625.

[7] Hiebert L.M., Liu J., Heparin protects cultured arterial endothelial cells from damage by toxic oxygen metabolites, *Atherosclerosis* 1990; 83: 47-51.

[8] Mandal A.K., Ping T., Caldwell S.J., Bagnell R., Hiebert L.M., Electron microscopic analysis of glucose-induced endothelial damage in primary culture: Possible mechanisms and prevention, *Histol. Histopathol* 2006; 21 : 941-950.

[9] Aryangat A.V., Gerich J.E., Type 2 diabetes: Postprandial hyperglycemia and increased cardiovascular risk, *Vascular Health and Risk* Management 2010; 6;145-155.

[10] Nosandini R., Tonolo G., Relationship between blood glucose control, pathogenesis and progression of diabetic nephropathy, *J. Am. Soc. Nephrol.* 2004;15 (Suppl): S1-S5.

[11] Mandal A.K., Hiebert L.M., Khamis H., Dglucose is linked to renal function changes in diabetes, *Diab Res ClinPract* 2011; 91: 190-194.

[12] McCance D.R., Hanson R.L., Charles M.A., Jacobsson L.T., Pettitt D.J., Bennett P.H., et al., Comparison of tests for glycated hemoglobin and fasting and two hour plasma glucose concentrations as diagnostic methods for diabetes, *BMJ* 1994; 308: 1323-1328.

[13] Rodbard H.W., Jellinger P.S., Davidson J.A., Einhorn D., Garber A.J., Grunberger G., et al., Statement by and American association of clinical endocrinologists American college of endocrinology consensus panel on type 1 and type 2 diabetes mellitus: An algorithm for glycemic control, *Endocr. Pract* 2009; 15, 540-559.

[14] Springberg P.D., Carrett LE. Jr., Thompson AL. Jr., Collins N.F., Lordon R.E., Robinson R.R., Fixed and reproducible orthostatic proteinuria: Results of a 20-year follow up study, *Ann. Intern Med.* 1982; 97: 516-519.

[15] Zatz R., Dunn B.R., Meyer T.W., Anderson S., Rennke H.G., Brenner B.M., Prevention of diabetic glomerulopathy by pharmacologic amelioration of glomerular capillary hypertension, *J. Clin. Invest* 1986; 77: 1925-1930.

[16] Lewis E.J., Hunsicker L.G., Bain R.P., Rohde R.D., The effect of angiotensin-converting enzyme inhibition on diabetic nephropathy. *N. Engl. J. Med 1993*; 329: 1456-1462.

[17] Berger J.R., Hedayati S., Renal replacement therapy in the elderly population, *Clin. J. Am. Soc. Nephrol.* 2012; 7: 1039-1046.

[18] Mandal A.K., Hiebert L.M., Renal protection in diabetes: Is it affected by glucose control or inhibition of the rennin-angiotensin pathway. *Clin. Nephrol* 2008; 69: 159-178.

[19] Weinger K., Beverly E.A., Barrier to achieving glycemic targets: Who omits insulin and why, *Diabetes Care* 2010; 33:450-452.

[20] Mandal, A.K., Neki N.S., Diabetes: Pragmatic therapy with a goal to preventing end stage kidney disease and dialysis, *Open Jour. Int. Med* 2011;1:80-92.

[21] Holman R.R., Pal S.K., Bethel M.A., Mathews D.R., Neil H.A., 10-year follow up of intensive glucose control in Type 2 diabetes, *N. Engl. J. Med* 2008; 359: 1577-1589.

[22] Palumbo P.J., The case for insulin treatment early in type 2 diabetes, *Clev. Clin. J. Med* 2004; 7: 385-405.

Chapter VII

Post Prandial Hyperglycemia: How Important Is Control of Postprandial Hyperglycemia in Diabetes

Abstract

Postprandial hyperglycemia is the most neglected component of the glycemic parameters ordered to diagnose and treat patients with diabetes. The reason is gaps of knowledge about the utility of postprandial glucose (PPG) among the professionals. Fasting blood glucose (FBG) and glycosylated hemoglobin (HbA1c) are the most publicized tests but the sensitivity of these tests are low. Thus, many patients who are labeled with Type 2 diabetes using the tests do not have diabetes. More important than the diagnosis is the relationship of PPG to outcome measures. Most clinical trials used FBG and HbA_1c for outcome measures. The preferred therapy is metformin, which predictably lowers HbA_1c. No clinical trials have been done to reveal if metformin lowers PPG levels. Strong evidence for that exists because despite the pre-ponderant use of metformin, the rate of diabetic complications is on the rise. Author's studies, which involve renal outcome, have shown promising results with insulin therapy, which predictably lowers PPG. Thus, it is important that we develop prospective studies with insulin versus oral antidiabetic agents in controlling postprandial hyperglycemia and determining its impact on outcome measures.

Diagnosis of Diabetes

Postprandial means after a meal; therefore, postprandial glucose (PPG) concentrations refer to plasma glucose concentration after a major meal. PPG is invalid after consuming tea and a piece of toast. In the western culture, breakfast is a favorite and major meal whereas in eastern cultures, lunch is a major meal. Because the absorption of food persists for 5-6 hours after a meal in both diabetic and non-diabetic individuals, the exact time to measure PPG concentration has not been determined. However, the optimal time for measurement of postprandial plasma glucose is 2 hours after a meal, generally approximating the peak value in patients with diabetes and providing a reasonable assessment of postprandial hyperglycemia. Specific conditions, such as gestational diabetes or pregnant women with diabetes, may benefit by testing at 1 hour after the meal [1].

Author always orders fasting and a 2-hour postprandial basic metabolic panel (BMP) for every patient. BMP is a composite laboratory test that provides glucose levels, renal functions tests with BUN, serum creatinine and the estimated glomerular filtration rate (eGFR), and electrolytes including Na+, K+, Cl-, CO2- and calcium.

It is not yet established what the normal 2hPPG is and what level of 2hPPG establishes the diagnosis of diabetes or diabetes mellitus (DM). The criteria used to determine diabetes was recommended by the National Diabetes Data Group (NDDG) in 1979 [2] and by the World Health Organization (WHO) in 1980 [3]. They are based on longitudinal studies conducted in the USA and the United Kingdom on people with variable degrees of glucose intolerance. These people were followed prospectively for diabetes complications, primarily retinopathy, as the end point. It was found that individuals whose 2hPPG was ≥ 200mg/dL (≥11.1mmol/L), even when their fasting glucose values were unequivocally normal were at the highest risk of developing diabetic complications. All other subjects, either those with impaired glucose tolerance [fasting glucose < 140mg/dL (<7mmol/L) and 2hPPG 140-199 mg/dL (<7-11mmol/L] or normal glucose tolerance [fasting glucose <140mg/dL (7mmol/L and 2hPPG <140 mg/dL (7mmol/L), were unlikely to develop complications. Thus, the criteria of glucose levels are important. They are not necessarily essential to determine the diagnosis but to determine the risk of developing the complications specific to diabetes [4]. In addition, virtually everyone with a fasting glucose value ≥140mg/dL also has a 2hPPG ≥ 200mg/dL. Thus, the fasting value is not needed to ascertain diabetes. Finally, 2hPPG is the key for detecting (and determining) diabetes [4].

Importance of Postprandial Hyperglycemia in Screening and Detection of Undiagnosed Diabetes

Screening can be interpreted as public health screening in the community, but also simply as testing for diabetes in the patients in the clinician's office. The 2-h postprandial glucose (2hPPG) is the most satisfactory screening method. Using a value of $\geq$ 200mg/dL, sensitivity is 97%; only 3% of individuals have 2hPPG < 200mg/dL and are considered to have diabetes attributable to fasting values $\geq$ 140g/dL only. Specificity is 100% because all non-diabetic individuals have 2-hPPG < 200mg/dL. The positive predictive value is also 100% because everyone with a 2hPPG > 200mg/dL is considered to have diabetes. Fasting blood glucose (FBG) is generally used for screening but it is an inadequate screening test. If a fasting value of $\geq$100mg (5.5mmol/L) was used as a cut off value for screening, sensitivity would be 83% and specificity would be 76%, but positive predictive value would be 21%; that is 4 of 5 individuals would not have diabetes. If the cutoff point was increased to a fasting value of $\geq$ 140mg/dL, sensitivity decreases significantly and only 31% of undiagnosed diabetes would be detected [4].

The validity of a screening test is usually measured in terms of four factors:

1. Sensitivity: The ability of the test to correctly identify people who have the disease
2. Specificity: The ability of the test to correctly identify people who do not have the disease
3. Positive predictive value: The proportion of people with positive test results who actually have the disease
4. Negative predictive value: The proportion of people with negative test results who actually do not have the disease.

Sensitivity is a measure of the false-negative rate (i.e. the number of negative results among people who have the disease), whereas specificity is a measure of the false-positive rate (i.e. the number of positive results among people who do not have the disease). The positive predictive value of a screening test depends primarily on the prevalence of disease in the population being screened; the higher the prevalence, the higher the positive predictive value.

Controversies in Understanding Postprandial Hyperglycemia and the Relationship of Postprandial Hyperglycemia to Complications

There are profound gaps in knowledge about postprandial hyperglycemia. Since the consensus conference on postprandial blood glucose by the American Diabetes Association in 2001, very little progress has been made in elucidating the importance of 2hPPG in determining the development and prevention of complications of diabetes. The reason is simple, few or no professionals order 2hPPG or 2hPPBMP. Author consistently orders 2hPPBMP for all patients: diabetes or non-diabetes office patients and has the most convincing data on 2hPPG and renal function changes. Also, we have the innovative data on glucose (2hPPG –FBG) to better understand the validity of 2hPPG relative to diabetic complications. In the past, the epidemiological and observational studies such as DCCT, the Stockholm diabetes study, Kumamoto's study, and UKPDS, relied predominantly on measures of chronic glycemia, such as HbA1c. No clinical trials ever addressed whether 2hPPG independent of other measure of glycemia, plays a unique role in the pathogenesis of diabetes – specific complication. Similarly, no clinical trial outside of studies in gestational diabetes has examined the need to treat postprandial glucose levels specifically to prevent complications [1]. Notably in the early stages of diabetes, when FBG and HbA1c are within acceptable ranges, postprandial hyperglycemia can cause macrovascular complications (such as myocardial infarction) and microvascular complications. In the United Kingdom prospective diabetes study (UKPDS) about 50% of the subjects had already experienced diabetic complications by the time they were first diagnosed with diabetes. A consistent body of data demonstrates a robust association between PPG and cardiovascular risk [5]. Large epidemiological studies have shown a continuous graded direct relation between the level of postchallenge glycemia and the risk for events, including coronary heart disease, stroke, sudden cardiac death, and peripheral vascular disease [6]. The worst problem with these previous studies is that no information is available about how these patients were treated and whether treatment minimized the severity of complications.

Renal Protection in Diabetes

The author and collaborators feel that lowering of blood glucose to near normal levels in diabetes is a reasonable thought. But realistically trying to lower blood glucose levels to normal levels with intensive insulin therapy is associated with a high risk of hypoglycemic reactions. Further, there is no evidence to indicate that keeping the glucose levels at normal levels will prevent cellular injury or repair any damage that has already been incurred. Therefore, the goal of adequate glycemic control is to keep 2hPPG at an optimal level (< 200mg/dL), which will not produce hypoglycemia. Hypoglycemia is a fearful experience that will distract patients to adhere to insulin injections. There is no yardstick available in the literature to determine optimal glycemic levels, which will confer renal protection. However, there is subtle evidence that 2hPPG > 200mg/dL is associated with a significant decrease of glomerular filtration rate; whereas keeping 2hPPG of < 200mg/dL gives rise insignificant changes in renal function [7]. In line with that valuable study, we have noted that elevation of glucose level > 200mg/dL at 2 hour post prandial period is associated with a discernible increase of serum creatinine (Scr) and a proportional decrease of eGFR compared to fasting glucose when sampled on the same day. The changes are not notable when 2hPPG rises < 200mg/dL. A patient is illustrated to that effect. An 80-year-old Canadian male came to the author's office as a self-referral for diabetes control. He is of average build, younger looking than his age, and very active. He gave a history of hypertension. He was treated with oral anti-diabetic agents and Lisinopril, which were discontinued and he was started on insulin therapy. He was admitted to a local hospital for shortness of breath. Myocardial infarction was considered but could not be documented. An office visit thereafter showed the following laboratory findings.

Table 1.

Glucose (mg/dL)		Scr (mg/dL)		eGFR (ml/min)	
F	2hPP	F	2hPP	F	2hPP
114	235	1.18	1.28	>60	58

dglucose (235-114) 121 mg/dL.

Dglucose was (235-114) 121mg/dL 24 hour urine protein was < 111mg and creatinine clearance 67.7ml/min. F = fasting 2hPP > 2 hour postprandial.

Author's patients are uniformly treated with a combination of Glargine insulin (Lantus®) or detemir (Levimir®) and fast acting insulin such as aspart (Novolog) or Novolin R or Humulin R. A few patients receive alpha glucosidase inhibitor (acarbose) or pioglitazone (Actos®). Author's patients do not receive angiotensin converting enzyme inhibitor (ACEI) or angiotensin receptor blocker (ARB) at any time. We have innovated d(delta) glucose (2hPPG-FBG) to increase the predictive value of glycemic control relative to renal function changes. We did the same equation relative to Scr and eGFR like dScr and deGFR(2hPPG eGFR-FBGeGFR). These are presented in Figure 1A and 1B.

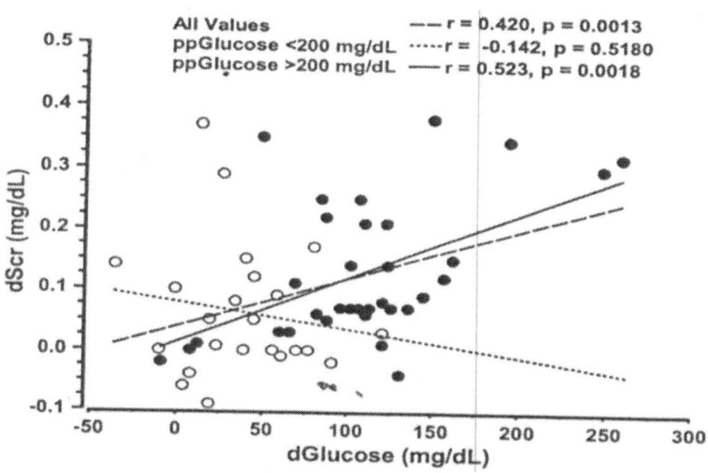

Figure 1A. Correlation of dScr (2hPP-F) with dglucose (2hPP=F). Correlation between dScr and dglucose and correlation coefficients and *p* values are shown for all 56 patients (dashed line, all data points), for patients whose 2hPP glucose is greater than 200 mg/dL (solid line, black circles, n+33) and for patients whose 2hPP glucose is less than 200 mg/dL (dotted line, open circles, n = 23).
Mandal et al. Diab Res Clin Pract 2011; 91: 190-194 reproduced with permission.

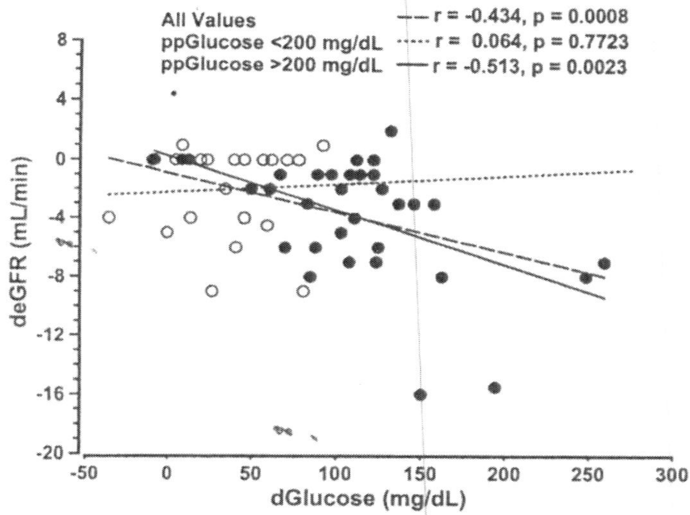

Figure 1B. Correlation of deGFR (2hPP-F) with dglucose (2hPP=F) Correlation between deGFR and dglucose and correlation coefficients and *p* values are shown for all 56 patients (dashed line, all data points), for patients whose 2hPP glucose is greater than 200 mg/dL (solid line, black circles, n = 33) and for patients whose 2hPP glucose is less than 200 mg/dL (dotted line, open circles, n = 23).
Mandal et al. Diab Res Clin Pract 2011; 91: 190-194 reproduced with permission.

Analysis of this study is based on a sample size of 56 patients, insuring reliable detection of important effects. In the initial observation, we documented that in patients whose 2hPPG is greater than 200mg/dL, for every 100mg/dL increase in dglucose, dScr increases by 0.11mg/dL and deGFR decreases by 3.73ml/min, while in patients whose 2hPPG < 200mg/dL for every 100mg/dL increase in d glucose little change is seen in dScr (-0.04mg/dL) or deFGR(+0.54ml/min). Average glucose and HbA_1c are poorly correlated with fasting renal function parameters [8]. The results of our most recent study (unpublished) are in agreement with the previous study thus confirming the validity of d glucose in ascertaining renal function changes.

Since we observed that renal function change is insignificant by keeping 2hPPG < 200mg/dL with intensive insulin therapy, we have examined the long-term effects of intensive glucose control on progression of renal function change in diabetes. We also reported that d glucose is more predictive of renal function change than 2hPPG. Our current study (unpublished) shows that d glucose above 50mg/dL relates significantly to renal function deterioration. Since d glucose is a derivative of 2hPPG, the higher the 2hPPG, the higher the d glucose, and the higher the serum creatinine. Our studies consistently demonstrate that intensive insulin therapy is associated with complete protection against end stage renal disease in diabetes. A complimentary adjuvant therapy is complete exclusion of ACEI/ARB drugs in diabetes. An important question can be asked to that effect: is the glucose level or the therapy important for renal protection in diabetes? We have already stated that both FBG and 2hPPG may remain elevated, but renal function change is minimal from one visit to the next or from the first to the last visit in those treated with insulin therapy. A major difference in therapy, as we have noted, is that metformin has slight or no effect on 2hPPG compared to insulin, which significantly lowers 2hPPG. Serum creatinine is significantly elevated over time in those treated with metformin compared to no or non-significant change in renal function in those treated with insulin.

Other investigators confirmed the importance of postprandial hyperglycemia. There is evidence that postprandial hyperglycemia, but no fasting hyperglycemia, independently predicts the occurrence of cardiovascular events [9].

The author has stated that there is no known threshold for glucose above which the risk for complications is higher than below the threshold. The Decode study [6] found exactly that. The Decode study [6] found that in subjects without a previous history of diabetes, there was no threshold for either a fasting or 2-hour postload glucose concentration above which would risk all causes or CVD death increased sharply. However, a gradually increasing relation between 2hPPG and CVD mortality was observed.

Other Therapeutic Paradigm

Once again, our study confirms that insulin treatment may not lower the 2hPPG appreciably but unequivocally confers renal protection as seen in our short-term and long-term studies. However, to date, there have been no prospective clinical trials evaluating the impact of improved postprandial hyperglycemia on long-term outcomes in patients with diabetes except renal protection in our prospective observational studies. Compared to traditional oral anti-diabetic agents such as metformin and glyburide, a-glucosidase inhibitors, including the meglitinide group of drugs, has been tested to treat postprandial hyperglycemia. The meglitinide analogues, including acarbose and miglitol, inhibit the alpha-glucosidase enzymes that line the brush border of the small intestine, interfering with hydrolysis of carbohydrates and delaying absorption of glucose and other monosaccharides. To lower postprandial glucose concentrations, these drugs must be taken with each meal. This group of drugs has been found to be useful in those who are noncompliant in diet control. These drugs are associated with distinct adverse effects. Unabsorbed carbohydrates cause abdominal pain, diarrhea, and flatulence due to osmotic effects and bacterial fermentation. Patients often feel embarrassed to go in public places because of flatulence and diarrhea and because of those side effects, some patients stop taking these groups of drugs. Beginning with low doses and increasing slowly can minimize these effects. Acarbose in high doses has been associated with moderate elevation in hepatic enzymes; miglitol has not. Author prescribes acarbose or miglitol in combination with insulin in patients in whom glucose control is difficult, despite high doses of insulin.

Pearl of Wisdom

Postprandial hyperglycemia is a fundamental issue in establishing the diagnosis of diabetes. Postprandial blood glucose above 200mg/dL (>11.1mmol/L) determines diabetes and the risk for developing complications. Pitifully no attention is paid in obtaining postprandial blood glucose because of the power of prevailing commercialism in diabetes care. Prevalent therapy in diabetes is a variety of oral antidiabetic agents, which lower fasting blood glucose and glycosylated hemoglobin (HbA_1c) but not postprandial glucose. No data is yet available to document that oral antidiabetic agents prevent foot ulcers, gangrene, or end stage renal disease requiring dialysis, the costliest therapy in diabetes care. Insulin therapy does it all. Oral antidiabetic agents are convenient to take thus they are satisfactory for the patients; hence, they come back to doctors again and again until they develop the catastrophic incident or more complications. Thus, patients should be educated to take insulin injections and avoid developing serious complications in lieu of experience of slight pain by insulin injection.

References

[1] American Diabetes Association Postprandial blood glucose. *Diab Care* 2001; 24: 775-778.

[2] National Diabetes Group classification and diagnosis of diabetes Mellitus and other categories of glucose intolerance. *Diabetes* 1979; 28: 1039-57.

[3] World Health Organization: *WHO Expert committee on diabetes Mellitus: Second Report.* Geneva, World Health Organization, 1980 (Tech Rep Serno 646).

[4] Harris MI. Undiagnosed NIDDM: clinical and Public Health Issues. *Diab Care* 1993; 16: 642-652.

[5] Cavalot, F, Petralli A, Traversa M et al., Postprandial blood glucose is a stronger predictor of Cardiovascular events than fasting blood glucose in Type 2 diabetes Mellitus. *J clin EndocrinolMetab* 2006; 91: 813-9.

[6] Decode study. Is the current definition of diabetes relevant to mortality risk from all causes and cardiovascular and non-cardiovascular disease. *Diab Care* 2003; 26:688-696.

[7] Nosadinin R, Tonolog. Relationship between blood glucose control, pathogenesis and progression of diabetic nephropathy. *J Am Soc Nephrol* 2004; 15 (suppl): S1-S5.

[8] Mandal Ak, Hiebert LM, Khamis H, dglucose relates to renal function changes in diabetes. *Res Clin Pract* 2011; 91: 190-194.

[9] Node K, Inove T. Postprandial hyperglycemia as an etiologic factor in Vascular failure cardiovascular Diabetology 2009; 8: 23. Open Access.

Chapter VIII

Pathophysiology and Prevention of End Stage Renal Disease in Diabetes Mellitus

Abstract

Renal failure whether acute renal failure (ARF), chronic renal failure (CRF) or end stage renal disease (ESRD) is not a mandate for dialysis therapy. Most commonly, ARF, CRF or ESRD is associated with the use of angiotensin converting enzyme inhibitor (ACEI), angiotensin receptor blocker (ARB) or a combination of both for treatment of proteinuria. A just published work reveals that diabetic patients treated with ACEI or ARB for 26 months showed eGFR reduction of 6.5 ± 0.4 ml/min per $1.73m^2$ compared to eGFR reduction of 2.1 ± 0.4 ml/min per $1.73m^2$ in another group but was treated additionally with pentoxifylline. Uncontrolled diabetes associated with osmotic diuresis, with volume depletion and low blood pressure, make diabetes patients very vulnerable to the hemodynamic effect of ACEI/ARB therapy. Thus, patients developed ARF when the hemodynamic effect was severe, or CKD with progression to ESRD when the hemodynamic compromise was persistent but less severe. Continuation of ACEI/ARB drugs in patients with diabetes and CKD results in decreased urine output and fluid overload giving rise to congestive heart failure (CHF) and severe anemia leading to a full blown picture of symptomatic uremia, thus warranting dialysis. This hasty progression of CKD with associated complications such as CHF and anemia is avoidable by not using ACEI/ARB therapy. Glucose control with insulin is an integral part of diabetes care. Adequate blood pressure control with antihypertensive drugs including beta blockers, calcium channel blockers or a combination is safe and effective in lowering blood pressure, which adds to renal preservation in diabetes. In some cases, a low dose of chlorthalidone adds to the control of blood pressure. Dialysis therapy should be considered as an accident and not a routine therapeutic approach for renal failure whether acute or chronic.

Nomenclature and Pathophysiology

Chronic renal failure (CRF) or chronic kidney disease (CKD) is generally non-reversible and often progressive. The term end stage renal disease (ESRD) is used to denote advanced CRF. The terms CRF and CKD will be used interchangeably throughout the chapter. Virtually all reports of ESRD refer to "treated" ESRD that is, patients who receive renal replacement therapy whether by dialysis or kidney transplant [1]. CKD is defined as the presence of kidney damage detected by proteinuria or decreased kidney function determined by the estimated glomerular filtration rate (eGFR) of < 60 ml/min for three or more months irrespective of the cause [2]. The five-stage classification, adopted by kidney disease outcomes is a quality initiative improving global outcomes (KDOQ1) although it is a bit lengthy and difficult to use in everyday practice. Most laboratories describe eGFR of > 60 ml/min as normal and of < 60 ml/min as renal failure. ESRD is defined as eGFR of < 15 ml/min [2, 3]. Diabetes or diabetic nephropathy is generally described as the most common cause of CKD and ESRD throughout the world including the USA [4-7]. Hypertension is second to diabetes as the most common cause of ESRD. Even in India where glomerular diseases are more prevalent than in the western world, diabetes stands out as the most common cause of ESRD [8]. Since no data is available with regard to causes of ESRD, from the majority of the countries, unresolved post infectious glomerulonephritis (GN), membranous GN, membranoprolferative GN and focal glomerular sclerosis appear to be other common causes of ESRD. 1gA nephritis is emerging as a common cause of ESRD worldwide. Less common causes of CKD include light chain nephropathy, myeloma kidney, ischemic nephropathy from bilateral mild to moderate renal artery stenosis, atheroembolic disease of the kidneys and chronic transplant nephropathy [9]. The glomerular filtration rate (GFR) is considered as the best overall indicator of renal function. GFR determination using creatinine clearance (crcl) is most commonly recommended in clinical practice. However, in order to obtain an accurate crcl, proper urine collection is important, but this is difficult to accomplish in some patients because of a poor understanding of the method of urine collection.

Accurate ways to measure GFR are by iothalamate clearance or insulin clearance, neither of which is obtainable in clinical practice. Therefore, clinicians have to settle with the use of crcl or eGFR using the abbreviated formula, which is essentially calculated from serum creatinine, taking into account age, gender and race [10]. CKD stages according to eGFR are shown.

MDRD Formula (eGFR)
Normal = > 60 ml/min/1.73m^2
Chronic kidney disease = < 60ml/min/1.73m^2
CKD stage 1< 60 > 50 ml/min/1.73m^2
CKD stage 2 < 50 > 40 ml/min/1.73m^2
CKD stage 3< 40 > 30 ml/min/1.73m^2
CKD stage 4< 30 > 20 ml/min/1.73m^2
CKD stage 5< 20 > 10 ml/min/1.73m^2
CKD stage 6 or ESRD< 10 ml/min/1.73m^2 (Medicare, USA)

Using the above definition the approximate prevalence of CKD is 2.5-11.2% of the adult population across Europe, Asia, North America, and Australia. In developed countries, age, hypertension, diabetes, increased body mass index and smoking are consistently associated with CKD.

Relationship of Proteinuria and Impact of Therapy on the Progression of Chronic Kidney Disease

Proteinuria in diabetic and non-diabetic renal disease is a prevalent issue in current medical practice and is associated with increasing pressure to treat proteinuria, including microalbuminuria, with ACEI/ARB or a combination of both groups of drugs. It is generally considered that reduction of proteinuria using the above drugs will delay progression of diabetic or non-diabetic nephropathy into ESRD.

In diabetes, proteinuria has been attributed to glomerular hyperfiltration, and by reducing glomerular hyperfiltration with ACEI/ARB therapy, proteinuria can be reduced and glomerular sclerosis can be mitigated. Other authors including the author himself refute the above hypothesis. A previous study found no benefit of treating microalbuminuria or proteinuria with ACEI therapy in diabetes. On the contrary, the authors of this study found progression of microalbuminuria to overt proteinuria in those who were treated with ACEI. Similarly, a previous study from this group showed that in diabetic patients with microalbuminuria, the risk of progression to overt proteinuria was reduced by improved glycemic control [11].

Other studies agree that adequate glycemic control (2hPP glucose < 200 mg/dl; HbA_1c < 7.5%) is fundamental to mitigation of progression of proteinuria and preservation of renal function. We have observed that the decrease in proteinuria with ACEI or ARB therapy is associated with parallel reduction in renal function suggesting that a decrease in proteinuria is related to a decrease of overall renal function. Two patients are illustrated to that effect (Tables 1 and 2).

Table 1. Effect of fosinopril on proteinuria and renal function in a 67-year-old African-American female with a 12-year history of diabetes

Date 1999-2006	24h Proteinuria (mg)	24 Crcl (ml/min)	Serum Creatinine (mg/dL)
October 17, 1999	160	125	0.8
Fosinopril 20 mg daily started			
November 9, 2000	88	90	0.9
December 8, 2002	142	81	1.0
February 18, 2004	5	55	1.1
Fosinopril discontinued			
July 15, 2004	151	96	1.0
January 20, 2005	417	76	1.0
April 7, 2005	215	86	0.9
June 8, 2006	257	70	0.7
December 11, 2006	< 150	80	1.0

Crcl = creatinine clearance.

As shown in Table 1, this 67 year African American female was prescribed fosinopril to reduce proteinuria of 160 mg per 24 hours. This is almost normal proteinuria because two-third of this proteinuria is tubular protein. After five years of fosinopril treatment, her proteinuria decreased to almost undetectable levels but with a parallel decrease in crcl of 50%. During this time period Scr increased slightly but was not noticeable. Fosinopril was discontinued, after which proteinuria returned with increase of crcl.

Table 2. Serially 24h proteinuria, BUN, and serum creatinine levels in a 59-year-old white female

Date	24-h Proteinuria (mg)	BUN (mg/dL)	Serum Creatinine (mg/dL)
June 25, 2005	5010		
September 30, 2005		45	4.1
October 2, 2005	3071	61	5.7

Home medication: glyburide, Lisinopril, amlodipine.
BUN increased by 16 mg/dL and serum creatinine increased by 1.6 mg/dL in 3 days.
Lisinopril was discontinued and bicarbonate infusion was started by the author. Author was an on-call nephrologist. However, the patient's regular nephrologist started her on hemodialysis treatment.

As shown in Table 2 this white female, age 59, was found to have heavy proteinuria (5010 mg per 24 hours) on June 25, 2005. She was prescribed Lisinopril 20mg po daily. In less than 4 months her proteinuria decreased by 2g per 24 hours but only at the expense of rapid decrease of renal function. Hence, both BUN and Scr increased sharply and her nephrologist placed her on hemodialysis treatment. Her nephrologist did not care to wait to find out about the recovery of renal function, which happens if Lisinopril is discontinued.

It is commonly believed that proteinuria adversely affects renal function. This is not true. It is true that heavy proteinuria signifies nephron damage but is not necessarily associated with progressive decline of renal function. Here is an example to that effect.

A white male, age 59, sought consultation with the author for heavy proteinuria in 2004. He had a kidney biopsy done before consultation with the author and after that he was placed on Lisinopril 20 mg po daily to reduce proteinuria. Proteinuria decreased so did renal function. Lisinopril was discontinued. Renal function worsened further for a short time then got better. Although proteinuria remained heavy renal function showed no or slight change. Definitely progressive deterioration of renal function was not noted. Details of proteinuria and renal function tests are presented in Table 3.

Table 3. Serially 24h proteinuria, creatinine clearance, and serum creatinine levels in a 59-year-old white male with lipoprotein nephropathy

Date 2004-2007	24h Proteinuria (mg)	24h Ccl/eGFR (ml/min)	Serum Creatinine (mg/dL)
December 15, 2004	8119	80	1.5
January 25, 2005	1901	NA	1.6
Lisinopril discontinued			
April 7, 2005	2920	96	1.5
August 15, 2005*	1144	77	1.7
Pentoxifylline 400 mg po twice daily			
November 7, 2005	1290	87	1.5
April 12, 2006	1316	104	1.3
Pentoxifylline reduced to 400 mg po once daily *			
January 19, 2007	ND	eGFR > 60	1.2
Dizziness; Flomax® changed to doxazosin 1 mg po once daily			
June 20, 2007	1853	105	1.3
July 27, 2007	2805	117.6	1.3
August 11, 2008	1949	104	1.3
April 9, 2009	1470	81	1.1
Medication: doxazosin 4 mg daily; metoprolol 25 mg daily; pentoxifylline 400 mg x 1 daily; allopurinol 150 daily; Lipitor® 20 mg daily; a proton pump inhibitor ® 20 mg daily			
January 11, 2010	5729	97.6	1.4
February 23, 2010	3337	82	1.3
September 30, 2010	2387	139.8/67.8	1.1
December 16, 2014	4696.5	120	1.37

ND = not done; NA = not available.

*= urinary frequency and Strangury associated with enlarged prostate. He was treated with Flomax® by a urologist. Subsequently, urinary symptoms were reduced to minimal.

Evidence from the older literature [12] before the availability of ACEI/ARB, as well as the author's own observations, indicate that proteinuria is not adverse to renal function. On the other hand, manipulation of proteinuria with ACEI or ARB therapy is associated with a steady decline of renal function. There is no discerning mechanism identified thus far by which ACEI/ARB can reduce proteinuria, except by reducing GFR.

Pentoxifylline, a methylxanthine derivative and non-specific phosphodiesterase inhibitor has been used to treat peripheral vascular disease for a long time. A previous study showed that pentoxifylline administration to patients with diabetes resulted in the reduction of clinical markers of glomerular and tubulointerstitial injury [13]. Thus, it may be worthy of trying pentoxifylline 1200 mg/day as in this study to reduce proteinuria.

Drugs Causing Chronic Kidney Disease (CKD) or End Stage Renal Disease (ESRD)

Drugs of concern here are angiotensin converting enzyme inhibitor (ACEI) and angiotensin receptor blocker (ARB). Unabated use of these groups of drugs are the most common cause of CKD in diabetes and the progression of CKD to ESRD. Published observations of the author attest to the commentary [14].

Other articles [15, 16], on the contrary, described these drugs as renoprotective. Based on the weight of these articles as well as other articles in line with these two articles, pharmaceutical companies who are producers of these groups of drugs have virtually gained authorative power to entice professionals to prescribe these drugs indiscriminately to patients with diabetes, hypertension, or other renal diseases to prevent progression of CKD into ESRD. State and Federal health care systems such as Medicare and Medicaid services (CMS) have endorsed these drugs as renal and cardio protective and were further influenced by pharmaceutical companies who have mandated the prescription of these drugs for diabetes and congestive heart failure. Thus, if a physician intentionally doesn't prescribe these drugs, like the author himself, they will receive lesser payment than those who will advocate these drugs. Author's observation determines that many physicians understand the high risk of ARF or CKD with the use of these drugs but they are unable to resist the pressure from CMS, hence they are forced to prescribe them. This approach has been unsuccessful as increasingly more patients are admitted into dialysis clinics over the years *(Figure 1)*.

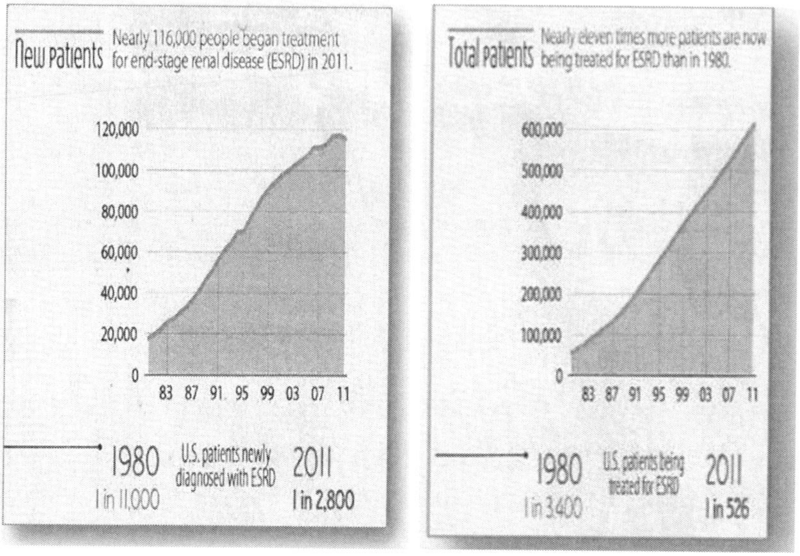

Figure 1. End Stage Renal Disease in United States.

For example, in 1980, 1 in 11,000 patients received renal replacement therapy as compared to 1 in 2,800 patients in 2011. The number of patients treated with renal replacement therapy in year 2011 was 11 times more than that in 1980. Why are patients with diabetes entering into dialysis clinics at a much faster rate now than they did before? The reason is that patients with uncontrolled diabetes because of inadequate or inappropriate treatment are often depleted of volume and electrolytes because of osmotic diuresis from heavy glucose load in the urine. This volume depletion makes the patients with uncontrolled diabetes most vulnerable to ACEI/ARB drugs giving rise to decreased renal perfusion and acute renal failure [17].

A patient is presented here to illustrate just that (Table 4)

After discontinuation of Lisinopril and by treatment with sodium bicarbonate infusion and insulin therapy his glucose control improved, and his renal function as shown by serum creatinine (Scr), and electrolytes returned to normal.

Acute kidney injury has been cited as a major factor that may contribute to development of ESRD in diabetes. Any episode of ARF was a risk factor for CKD stage 4 (hazard ratio 3.56); each ARF episode doubled that risk [18].

Further, aggressive blood pressure lowering treatment approaches with ACEI/ARB drugs may contribute to ARF episodes and enhance the CKD progression as described here [19].

Table 4. Serial Laboratory studies in a 59-year-old African American male with a long history of diabetes mellitus. Admitted to hospital for acute renal failure

Date 2005	Glucose (F) (mg/dL)	BUN (mg/dL)	Scr (mg/dl	Na^+ (mEq/l)	K^+ (mEq/l)	CO_2 (mEq/l)
Aug 18	302	76	7.4	126	5.9	15
Hospital admission: Lisinopril discontinued						
Aug 19	274	80	8.2	*127*	5.0	17 (pH 7.31, base excess -7.7)
Normal saline with 3 ampoules of sodium bicarbonate infusion started. Regular insulin given subcutaneously.						
Aug 20	249	68	2.2	133	5.6	18
Aug 21	196	22	0.8	139	4.2	32
Aug 22	186	10	0.8	140	3.8	33
Discharged from hospital						

F = fasting, BUN = blood urea nitrogen, Scr = serum creatinine.

Data from the United States ESRD program serves as a testimonial to the fact that ACEI/ARB drugs have paved the path to ESRD, requiring dialysis (Table 5) and placing the burden of this costly therapy on the health care system [7].

Table 5. Yearly number of patients in end stage renal disease (ESRD) dialysis program in the US

Year	ESRD-Dialysis Number of patients)
1978	14,000
1986	32,000
1993	ACEI entered the market
1994	65,000
1998	75,000 ARB entered the marked
2006	354,754
2011	616,000
2020 (projected)	750,000

It is evident that inadequate glycemic control, often with a suboptimal dose of insulin or most commonly with no insulin therapy or the use of ineffective insulin (70/30 mixtard, cloudy insulin) combined with oral anti-diabetic drugs and over enthusiastic use of ACEI/ARB drugs to reduce proteinuria is the main road for progression of indolent CKD to symptomatic ESRD [20].

Prevention of ESRD in Diabetes Mellitus

Given the background of expectant pathophysiology of ESRD, prevention of ESRD is attainable. Progression of CKD into ESRD can be minimized or abrogated in patients with DM by paying full attention to glycemic control and avoiding the use of ACEI/ARB. In a recent article on healthcare costs in people with diabetes and their association with glycemic control and kidney function the authors noted that the cost of caring for people with diabetes is substantial and is associated with suboptimal glycemic control, abnormal kidney function and proteinuria [21].

For those with DM, whose random glucose or 2hPPG is > 200 mg/dL (> 11.1 mmol/L) insulin is the cornerstone of therapy. Our experimental studies reinforce the clinical studies emphasizing that insulin therapy reverses toxic effects of high glucose on endothelial cells, which translates into prevention of clinical complications [22].

It is recommended that insulin therapy begin with long acting insulin. There are two types of very potent long acting insulin preparations available: Insulin Glargine (Lantus®) and insulin detemir (Levemir®). A recombinant DNA analog of human insulin (Lantus or detemir) forms microprecipitates in subcutaneous tissues, delaying its absorption and prolonging its duration of action. There are no peak blood insulin concentrations, thus mimicking continuous infusion of rapid acting insulin from a subcutaneous pump. Both Glargine and detemir insulin have a similar onset of action of about 4 hours, reaching a peak effect in 6-8 hours. The effect decreases after 12 hours. Author routinely recommends Glargine or detemir 25 units each, after breakfast and dinner (12 hours apart) with a gradual increase in dosage to maintain 2hPPG < 200mg (<11.1 mmol/L). Notably Glargine or detemir insulin taken twice daily has made a big difference in attaining satisfactory glycemic control and stability of renal function over time among the author's patients seen in the office and in the hospital [23].

In addition, patients who are non-compliant in diet or who are obese will require additional fast acting insulin in the form of aspart (Novolog®) or Lispro (Humalog®), Novolin R or Humulin R to control the glycemic excursions. A common recommendation is to take 10-15 units before each meal and a fourth dose at bedtime preferably using a standard sliding scale. There are three types of sliding scales: low, standard, or high dose.

Fingerstick Glucose range mg/dL	**Low Regular Insulin Units**	**Standard Regular Insulin Units**	**High Regular Insulin Units**
150-200	2	4	6
201-250	4	8	10
251-300	6	12	14
301-350	8	16	18
351-400	10	20	22
>400	Call physician		

Glargine or detemir insulin is expensive and may not be universally available. In lieu of these products, NPH insulin, every 12 hours, or a combination of Humulin N and Humulin R every 12 hours may prove to be effective.

Monitoring of Blood Glucose Control

Monitoring of blood glucose by finger stick practices on a daily basis by the patients themselves is an integral part of diabetes care. The most important glucose level to monitor is the post-meal surges. Glucose levels run like peaks and valleys. Lantus or Levemir twice daily will maintain the valleys. Peak glucose levels need to be controlled by fast-acting insulin as already stated. Glucose monitoring at home is a tedious job but as long as the patients feel well and don't develop the complications, they realize the value of glucose monitoring and taking insulin injections and thus remain committed to this responsibility.

Additional anti-diabetic agents: Two oral anti-diabetic agents including acarbose and or pioglitazone (Actos®) are prescribed occasionally in those where glycemic control remains difficult. Pioglitazone is an insulin sensitizer and thus promotes glycemic control. Usual dose is 15-30 mg per day. Swelling may be seen in the lower extremities. Acarbose is described in Chapter 9.

Control of Hypertension

Blood pressure control is additive to glycemic control in accomplishing the prevention of diabetic complications. A beta-blocker, calcium channel blocker, sympathetic inhibitor, or vasodilator drugs are efficacious and safe. A combination of two to three drug classes may be used to maintain effective blood pressure control. ACEI/ARB drugs are excluded in the author's practice

Blood pressure control is the goal, not the type of drugs used. In resistant cases use of diuretics such as 25 to 50 mg/day chlorthalidone effectively lowers blood pressure. In hypertensive patients with reduced GFR, neither amlodipine nor Lisinopril was found to be superior to chlorthalidone in reducing the development or 50% or greater decrease in GFR [24].

Pearl of Wisdom

There is abundant evidence including that of authors that treatment of diabetes with adequate doses of insulin prevents development and or progression of microvascular and macrovascular complications. Manipulation by oral antidiabetic agents alone to enhance endogenous insulin release or increase insulin sensitivity results in exhaustion of the beta cells, thus changing, over the years, an easily controllable glycemic state into a pathological uncontrollable glycemic state. Similarly, using ACEI/ARB drugs to reduce proteinuria results in ARF, CKD, and progression of CKD into ESRD. Thus, this type of practice must be abandoned. Glycemic control with insulin reduces proteinuria thus insulin is the cornerstone of therapy in diabetes. Patients must take responsibility of their care hand in hand with the professionals. Both parties must be unified to achieve only one goal, which is to learn to cope with diabetes yet thrive and not develop complications, such as end stage kidney failure [25].

References

[1] Eggers PW. Has the incidence of end stage renal disease in the USA and other countries stabilized. *CurrOpin Nephrol Hypertens* 2011; 20: 241-5.

[2] James M, Hemmelgara BR, Tonelli M. Early recognition and prevention of chronic kidney disease. *Lancet* 2010; 375: 1296-309.

[3] KDOQ1 Clinical practice guidelines for the evaluations and management of chronic kidney disease. *Kidney Int* (Suppl) 2012; 3-5.

[4] US Renal Data System 2011.

[5] Colins AJ, Foley RN, Chavers B, et al. United States Renal Data System 2011 Annual Data Report: Atlas of chronic kidney disease & end-stage renal disease in the United States. *AmJ Kidney Dis* 2012; 59(Suppl): e1-420.

[6] Atkins RC, Zimmet P. World Kidney Day 2010; Diabetic Kidney disease-act now or pay later. *AmJ Kidney Dis* 2010; 5: 205-8.

[7] Couser WG, Remuzzi G, Mends S, Tonelli M. The contribution of chronic kidney disease to the global burden of major non-communicable diseases. *Kidney Int* 2011; 80: 1258-970.

[8] Rajapurkar MM, John GT, Kirpalani AL et al. What do we know about chronic kidney disease in India First report of Indian CKD registry *BMC Nephrol* 2012; 13: 10 (open access).

[9] Mandal AK, Hiebert LM Pathophysiology and prevention of end stage renal disease in diabetes mellitus, *J Endocrinol Diab Mellitus* 2014; 2: 101-108.

[10] Woodhouse S, Batten W, Hendrick H, Malek PA. The glomerular filtration rate: an important test for diagnosis, staging and treatment of chronic kidney disease. *Lab Med* ; 37: 244-6.

[11] Ficociello IH, Perkins BA, Silva KH et al. Determinants of progression from microalbuminuria to proteinuria in patients who have type 1 diabetes and are treated with angiotensin – converting enzyme inhibitors. *Clin J Am Soc Nephrol* 2007; 2: 461-9.

[12] Schieppati A, Mosconi L, Pema A, et al. Prognosis of untreated patients with idiopathic membranous nephropathy N. *Engl J Med* 1993; 329: 85-9.

[13] Navarro-Gonzalez JF, Nora-Femandez C, deFuentes MM, et al. Effect of pentoxifylline on renal function and urinary albumin excretion in patients with diabetic kidney disease: the Predian Trial J. *Am Soc Nephrol* 2015; 26: 220-229.

[14] Mandal AK, Hiebert LM, Renal protection in diabetes: is it affected by glucose control or inhibition of the renin angiotensin path way? *Clin Nephrol* 2008; 69: 169-74.

[15] Lewis EJ, Hunsicker LG, Baui RP, Rode Rd. The effect of angiotensin converting enzyme inhibition on diabetic nephropathy. The collaborative study group N. *Engl J Med* 1993; 329: 1456-62.

[16] Brenner BM, Cooper ME, dezee UMD et al. Effect of Iosartan on renal and cardiovascular outcomes in patients with type 2 diabetes and nephropathy. *N. Eng J Med* 2001; 354: 861-9.

[17] Schoolworth AC, Sica DA, Ballernan BJ, *Wilcox CS Renal consideratins in angiotensin converting enzyme therapy circ* 2001; 104: 1985-91.

[18] Thakkar CB, Christianson A, Hammelfard J, Leonard AC, Acute kidney injury episodes and chronic kidney disease risk in diabetes mellitus clin *J Am Soc Nephrol* 2011; 6: 2567-72.

[19] Onuibo MA, Can Ace inhibitor and angiotensin receptor blockers be detrimental in CKD patients, *Nephron ClinPract* 2011; 118: C407-19.

[20] Suissa S, Huchinson T, Broph KM, Kezouh A Ace inhibitor use and the long term risk of renal failure in diabetes. *Kidney Int* 2006; 9: 913-9.

[21] McBrien KA, Manns BJ, Chui B et al. Healthcare cost in people with diabetes and their association with glycemic control and kidney function. *Diab Care* 2013; 36: 1172-80.

[22] Mandal AK, Ping T, Caldwell SJ et al. Electron microscopic analysis of glucoseinduced endothelial damage in primary cell culture. Possible mechanism and prevention *HistolHistopathol* 2006; 21: 941-50.

[23] Mandal AK, Neki NS Diabetes: a pragmatic therapy with a goal to prevent end stage kidney disease and dialysis *OJ M* 2011; 1: 80-92.

[24] Rahman M, Pressel S, Davis BR et al. Renal outcomes in high risk hypertensive patients treated with an angiotensin converting enzyme inhibitor or a calcium channel blocker vs. a diuretic (ALLHAT) *Arch Intern Med* 2005; 165: 936-6.

[25] Mandal AK Frequent office visits of patients with chronic kidney disease is aprelude to prevention of dialysis. *World J Nephrol* 2014; 3: 1-5.

Chapter IX

Pragmatic Therapy of Diabetes with Insulin: Gift of Life for Diabetes

Abstract

Although diabetes mellitus (DM) or sugar diabetes was identified centuries ago, it was not known why this metabolic disorder develops until JR Macleod and Frederick Banting made the discovery. DM is due to deficiency of insulin produced by beta cells of the pancreas. Before this discovery and its application around 1921, many people with this disorder died from diabetic coma. Thus, insulin made a milestone in the treatment of DM, in the early part of the 20th century and it is the same today. However, commercialism prevails in the care of DM with too much twist in the therapy. With prevalent use of oral anti-diabetic agents, which lower blood sugar levels but do not confer the benefit insulin did and still does. Thus, although patients are not dying from diabetic coma because of insulin but they are developing a whole gamut of complications, which have increased the morbidity and mortality in patients with DM. Thus the emphasis of this chapter is to resurge the use of insulin as a gift of life for patients with DM and may permit a healthy and active life for them.

Background of Discovery of Insulin and Its Application in Treating Diabetes

Although ancient Egyptians in 1500BC recognized diabetes or sugar diabetes, the real entity was not established until 1921 when Frederick Banting of the University of Toronto, Canada successfully treated a patient with insulin prepared from a pancreatic extract. In the autumn of 1918, a 15-year-old female developed polyuria, and complained of weakness, leg and back pain, and insomnia. In March 1919 these symptoms became more severe. The appetite became excessive and there was some pruritus. Body weight was progressively decreasing and glucose in urine was discovered. She came under the care of Banting on August 16, 1922 and showed emaciation, dry skin, slight edema of the ankles and thin and brittle hair. She was unable to walk and weighed 45 pounds. Insulin treatment was started immediately. Insulin was given 15 to 30 minutes before the morning and evening meals. A sufficient amount was given to keep the urine free of sugar. The diet was increased daily. On this treatment, she rapidly gained strength and soon was able to take on vigorous exercise. Weight increased from 45 to 105 pounds in the first six months. In June of 1925, she was in the best of health and in her words "never felt better in all my life" weight was 134lbs. The insulin required to keep her urine sugar free was reduced to about one-third [1] *Frederick Banting received the Nobel Prize in Medicine on September 15, 1925.*

Prevailing Commercialism Hindering Treatment of Diabetes with Insulin

Given the discovery of insulin's efficacy for treating diabetes, unfortunately therapy for diabetes has taken a different turn. This turn for the worse has been made possible by the influence of commercialism on our medical practices. Commercialism seems to prevail in "Diabetes care" more than any other illness and is orchestrated by drug companies in collaboration with professionals, which sadly promote profit over patients. Prevailing commercialism consists of promoting oral anti-diabetic drugs instead of insulin as a first line therapy for diabetes. This commercialism seems to be magnified by greedy industry and different medical societies. The roles of some politicians who are profoundly influenced by industries to advance their avarice; the often ridiculous reimbursement by Medicare that is not sufficient to pay their office expenses; and the failure of the private sector to create a system of health care that is not filled with greed, but barely meets the medical needs of all patients. The good doctor will, when the time is right, try to explain these important peripheral matters to their patients because the profession of medicine itself is seriously threatened by powerful corporate and political forces that do not understand the benefit of the patients and goals of the medical profession. In this regard, doctors need the help of their patients. But to restate, when a good doctor sees a patient, he or she tries at that time to help the patient despite the numerous obstacles that interfere with such an effort. We have persistently studied the aphorisms and writing of Sir William Osler, Paul D White, Eugene A Stead, Paul Beeson, and many other time-tested doctors. The author himself had the opportunity to spend some time with Dr. Eugene Stead. The messages left by these great physicians give us a glimpse of the best thinkers in the profession of medicine from antiquity to the present time. We learned from them that it was the type of service they rendered that established them as trustworthy in the minds of the patients who came to them for medical care. They all emphasized in their own unique way, that the best doctors manage the sick person's general response to a disease as well as the patient's specific reaction to the disease itself [2].

The author himself is a kind of good doctor described in reference number 2. A great conviction of the author is that in the office patients come first.

Therapy for Diabetes with Insulin

Compliance of the patients and attention of the professionals must work hand in hand to achieve the most benefit in diabetes care. It is imperative that we strive for early detection and treatment of diabetes mellitus (DM), so that complications can be averted. Treatment of complications is costly; therefore, current huge health care costs for DM can be reduced with early detection and treatment of DM. In 2009, cost of diabetes care among the Medicare eligible population was US $45 billion. Notwithstanding increasing awareness of diabetes; adequate funding for diabetes research, and the plethora of oral medication to treat diabetes, complication rates are showing no sign of decreasing. Here is an example: the Los Angeles Times as of March 22, 2009 reported that over the last 15 years, the US rate of foot amputations from complications of diabetes has soared, approaching 100,000 annually, according to studies and government statistics. To that effect, both parties are responsible. Professionals are not emphasizing adequate glucose control with insulin therapy. A recent report indicates that only 17% of patients with DM take insulin. Another 17% of patients with DM take a combination of insulin and oral agents, whereas 54% of diabetes patients are treated with oral agents. A 2004-2006 National Health Interview Survey is identical to the previous report as already stated. Despite availability of a variety of insulin preparations, good glucose control is unachieved. The lack of success is mainly due to lack of diet control and irregularities or refusal to take prescribed doses of insulin. The worst part of diabetes care is non-compliance in adhering to prescribed diet and insulin therapy. On the other hand, compliance of the patient and support system in following prescribed diet and insulin therapy along with better understanding of the seriousness of diabetes complications without insulin treatment and taking full responsibility of the care along with the professionals will go long way in averting the complications and staying healthy.

Here is an example of great compliance of the support system in rigidly following medical advice, which has made it possible for healthy living of this 73-year-old white male. He and his wife are residents of Montana, a northern state of the USA, and they live in Florida during the winter months. He was first seen in March 2014 by the author in consultation in a local hospital and thereafter was followed regularly in one of the author's offices. In March 2014, he was found very lethargic and poorly conversing. He was noted to have uncontrolled diabetes and acute or chronic renal failure. He was treated with oral anti-diabetic agents consisting of glipizide and a DPP-4 inhibitor and angiotensin receptor blocker losartan. These therapies were discontinued and he was started on detemir insulin (Levemir) 15 units after breakfast and dinner. Laboratory studies during hospital stay are shown in Table 1. After discharge, he was seen in author's office in April 2014. Medications consisted of detemir insulin 15 units after breakfast and dinner. Losartan 50mg daily, paroxetine 20mg daily, ferrous sulfate 300mg PO TID, DPP-4 inhibitor (onglyza®) 5mg daily, glipizide 10mg daily, furosemide 20mg PO as required and spironolactone 25mg PO as required.

Author's action was to discontinue glipizide and DPP-4 inhibitor and angiotensin receptor blocker (ARB) Losartan. Continue insulin detemir (Levemir®) 20 units after breakfast and dinner, and hydralazine PO 25mg BID was added. His next visit was in November 2014. Medications consisted of Novolin N 25 units morning and evening (could not afford Levemir), calcitriol 0.25mcg daily, ferrous sulfate as before, Vitamin C 500mg daily, dipyridamole

75mg 2 tablets morning and evening, hydralazine 25mg PO BID. He did his laboratory. The results are shown in Table 2.

Table 1. Day 1 of Hospital Admission

	Glucose (mg/dL)	BUN (mg/dL)	Scr (mg/dL)	eGFR (ml/min)	Hb (g/dL)
(Postprandial)	336	33	2.01	35	8.1

Ser = serum creatinine
Hb = Hemoglobin

Table 2.

	Glucose (mg/dL)	BUN (mg/dL)	Scr (mg/dL)	eGFR (ml/min)	Hb (g/dL)
Fasting	99	22	1.35	52	10.6
2hPP	130	22	1.23	58	

Urinalysis both periods were negative for glucose and protein.

Glucose control has improved to normal levels with insulin. Renal function has improved to near normal levels, as well as hemoglobin levels. All these improvements are due to insulin therapy and exclusion of the use of ARB drugs, Losartan. Author's action at this time was to discontinue dypyridamole as an additional cause of anemia and double the dosage of iron. His next visit was in January 2015. He is conversing much and feels as happy as his wife. His medications were same as in the previous visit except dipyridamole. He did his laboratory. The results are shown in Table 3.

Table 3.

	Glucose (mg/dL)	BUN (mg/dL)	Scr (mg/dL)	eGFR (ml/min)	Hb (g/dL)
Fasting	97	20	1.40	53	10.7
2hPP	134	20	1.2	>60	ND

Serum ferritin 374ng/ml stool occult.
Blood x3 were negative.

Glucose control is normal with Novolin N 25 units twice daily. Blood pressure was 110/70 mmHg. Postprandial renal function is normal thus the goal is met. Hemoglobin is still low but increasing. However, iron reserve is normal and there was no evidence of occult gastrointestinal bleeding. Author's action was to continue current therapy.

Rationale of Intensive Insulin Therapy

Glucose levels in a subject who is not diabetic are

- After overnight fasting less than 126mg/dL (7mmol/L), better is less than 100mg/dL (5.5mmol/L)
- 2 hours after an unrestricted breakfast or lunch (not tea and toast or salad and soup) less than 200mg/dL (<11.1mmol/L), better is ≤140mg/dL (<7.7mmol/L)
- In subject with established diabetes but untreated: overnight, fasting glucose can be over 200mg/dL (>11mmol/L) and 2 hours after breakfast or lunch can go as high as 400 or 500mg/dL (22.2-27.7mmol/L). The classification of Type 1 and Type 2 diabetes is not used anywhere in this book because the classification sheds no light in glycemic control or prevention strategy.

People with established diabetes whose blood glucose levels are higher than 200mg/dL (>11.1mmol/L) without treatment with insulin are at a high risk to develop complications acutely or in a protracted (chronic) fashion. It is important to remember that while acute complications reverse with intensive insulin therapy, chronic complications do not necessarily reverse even with intensive insulin therapy.

Acute complications of diabetes are diabetic ketoacidosis and diabetic coma. These are discussed briefly in chapter 4: complications of diabetes. In this chapter glycemic control with intensive insulin therapy and blood pressure control with anti-hypertensive drug therapy with exclusion of angiotensin converting enzyme inhibitor (ACEI) and ARB drugs will be emphasized. However, before reading on the therapy, it is important for the readers to know some fundamentals of therapy, which perhaps may make them feel comfortable to resort to the therapies presented here.

Thus, the chronic complications of diabetes are reiterated here and how do these complications develop from a pathobiological standpoint? The microvascular system is singularly affected and the vascular endothelial cells are the targets for serious damage by high circulatory glucose milieu. These chronic complications are below, but not in any particular order:

- Retinopathy leading to impaired vision
- Nephropathy leading to end stage renal disease (ESRD) and dialysis
- Unhealed foot ulcer or gangrene of toes or feet and amputation
- Sexual dysfunction
- Coronary heart disease leading to myocardial infarction and sudden death
- Neurogenic bladder leading to urinary retention and recurrent urinary tract infection
- Gastroparesis and paralytic ileus leading to recurrent vomiting, diarrhea, loss of nutrition and cachexia.

Thus when patients present to a doctor's office with one complication, careful examination reveals additional complications. Variable degrees of renal function impairment are common accompaniments of many of the diabetic complications listed above. The renal failure most commonly defined by eGFR<60ml/min is not necessarily and entirely due to uncontrolled diabetes but more often due to therapy.

An important question is about the threshold of glucose level above which complications are likely to develop and below which complications are unlikely to develop. No definite answer is available to that effect. The reason is most outcome studies used glycosylated hemoglobin (HbA_1c) as the only glycemic parameter to validate the results. However, studies from Europe and other countries used 2h postprandial glucose above 200mg/dL to determine cardiovascular morbidity and mortality. These are detailed in chapter 7: Postprandial hyperglycemia. Here is a hypothetical question and fundamental laboratory research of the author is presented to clarify the hypothesis. The hypothesis is, if glucose particles are injurious why doesn't a normal glucose level (70-99mg/dL or 4.4-5.5mmol/L) produce endothelial cell (Ecs) damage, but does so when Ecs are treated with high glucose (above 200mg/dLor 11.1mmol/L). However, Ecs damage is largely mitigated when Ecs are treated with high glucose simultaneously with insulin in the culture plate [3].

Thus, this research finding of the author validates the clinical scenario that insulin treatment prevents renal failure and perhaps other diabetes complications. However, it should be stressed at this point that all author's patients are treated with insulin and they all are living a complication-free life.

The most important therapy for diabetes is obviously replacement therapy, which is insulin. Early insulin therapy with resultant satisfactory glucose control appears to spare or delay beta-cell damage and might even spare beta-cell function. Glucose control can be graded into three categories, according to this study [4].

2-hour postprandial glucose levels: can be easily obtained by ordering 2-hour postprandial basic metabolic panel (BMP) after eating a normal breakfast or lunch, whichever is patient's preferred meal.

- Satisfactory = < 200mg/dL (<11.1mmol/L)
- Fair = 200-300mg/dL (11.1-16.6mmol/L)
- Poor = >300mg/dL (>16.6mmol/L)

Thus, satisfactory glucose control and frequent office visits to maintain the glucose control and adequate blood pressure and electrolyte and acid-base controls are prerequisites to prevention of complications strategy [5].

Principle of Insulin Therapy

A variety of insulin preparations are available in the market. Short (fast) acting, intermediate acting, and long acting. It is recommended that insulin therapy begin with long-acting insulin. There are two types of long-acting insulin available.

Insulin Glargine (Lantus®) and detemir (Levemir®) A recombinant DNA analog of human insulin, forms microprecipitates in subcutaneous tissue, delaying its absorption and prolonging its duration of action. Both have similar onset of action in about 4 hours and reach peak action in 8-9 hours. Effect decreases after 12 hours. There is no data to support or refute that either Lantus or Levemir will be effective for 24 hours in those with normal kidney function. Author prefers Lantus because he has more experience with that product. While Lantus or Levemir should be prescribed after breakfast and dinner (12 hours apart) in those with normal kidney function, once daily after breakfast is appropriate in those with reduced kidney function. Author typically prescribes 25 units after breakfast and dinner at the outset and increases dosage to achieve satisfactory glucose control. Although in some patients Lantus or Levemir alone can be used to achieve glycemic control and stabilize kidney function, many other patients will need coverage of fast acting or regular insulin coverage.

Fast-acting Insulins

1. Insulin aspart (Novolog®)
2. Insulin Lispro (Humolog®)
3. Novolin®
4. Humulin®

While aspart or lispro are very rapid acting (action starts within 20 minutes), Humulin or Novolin R are fast and action starts within 30-40 minutes.

Intermediate-acting

1. NPH (Neutral protamine Hagedorn)
2. Novolin N
3. 70/30 mixed insulin

NPH is uncommonly used in the USA; it may be different in other countries. A combination of Novolin R and Novolin N is effective in achieving glycemic control but the author is unsure about the efficacy of mixed insulin. The mixed insulin preparations are turbid, which decreases efficacy, thus the author does not recommend that insulin. Remember, insulin must be water-colored to be efficacious.

Satisfactory Glucose Control: Insulin Therapy

For patients with 2h postprandial or random glucose of less than 200mg/dL, the author recommends a trial of diet control, avoid excesses (buffet lunch or dinner, parties) and regular exercise to reduce weight if overweight or maintain baseline weight. Author does not recommend oral anti-diabetic agents as they reduce fasting blood glucose and HbA_1c but not 2h postprandial glucose, which is critical in development and progression of complications [6, 7].

Here is an isolated example of effect of insulin in lowering all the glycemic parameters: fasting glucose, 2-h postprandial glucose, and HbA_1c. Metformin even in large doses is ineffective compared to insulin.

A 54-year-old Cambodian female gave long history of diabetes and was treated with metformin 1000mg twice daily. The results are shown in Table 4.

Table 4. First office visit October 2010

	Glucose (mg/dL)	BUN (mg/dL)	Scr (mg/dL)	eGFR (ml/min)	HbA_1c %
Fasting	132	17	0.61	103	10.4
2hPP	292	ND	ND	ND	

At this visit, based on uncontrolled 2h postprandial blood glucose, metformin was discontinued and she was started on Glargine insulin (Lantus) 25 units subcutaneously after breakfast and after dinner (12 hours apart).

It should be noted that metformin didn't affect HbA_1c or 2h postprandial glucose.

Her next office visit was in February 2011. The laboratory is shown in Table 5.

Table 5.

	Glucose (mg/dL)	BUN (mg/dL)	Scr (mg/dL)	eGFR (ml/min)	HbA_1c%
Fasting	113	21	0.56	113	7.9
2hPP	204	19	0.60	104	ND

ND = Not done.
Scr = Serum Creatinine.
PP = Postprandial.

Lantus insulin effectively reduced fasting and 2hPP glucose levels, and HbA_1c and improved renal function.

Adversary to diabetes care is by not prescribing insulin to control hyperglycemia. Here is an outstanding example to that effect.

A 52-year-old African American male had his first office visit with the author in the latter part of December 2014. Before this office visit, he was admitted to a local hospital where he was living in February 2014. He was found to be a diabetic and treated with regular insulin during the hospital stay. Lisinopril was increased from 20mg/day to 40mg/day. Laboratory results upon admission and during hospital stay are shown in Table 6.

Table 6.

	February 27 2014 (Fasting)	March 5 (Fasting)
Glucose (mg/dL)	206	199
Serum Creatinine (mg/dL)	3.24	4.48
BUN (mg/dL)	37	54
eGFR (ml/min)	24.6	16.9
Na/K (mmol/L)	139/4.0	133/3.7

He was discharged from the hospital and followed by a primary care physician. He did not receive insulin after discharge from the hospital until he reported to the author's office.

He gave history of uncontrolled diabetes, which was first detected in year 2002. He was treated with metformin 1000mg PO daily. He also gave history of hypertension. Medications at this visit included: hydralazine 25mg x 3 TID, clonidine 0.1mg x 2 TID, atenolol 50mg daily, Lisinopril 40mg daily, doxazosin 2mg x 2daily calcitriol 0.25mcg daily, amlodipine 10mg daily, furosemide 40mg daily, simvastatin 40mg daily, Humulin N 10 units subcut at bed time just started.

On examination, he showed slight edema, blood pressure was 120/80 mttg. A limited laboratory done in early December 2014 showed random glucose of 421mg/dL (23.3mmol/L), serum creatinine of 3.14mg/dL and eGFR of 25ml/min. BUN was 53mg/dL. Hemoglobin 9.g/dL.

Assessment: uncontrolled diabetes, chronic kidney disease (CKD) stage 4, and anemia probably due to CKD and Lisinopril. Also, he showed low vitamin D Level.

Author's action included 1) Discontinue Lisinopril 2) reduce atenolol to 25mg/ PO daily 3) start glargine insulin (Lantus) 25 units after breakfast and 25 units after dinner 4) increase Humulin N 10 units before each meal 5) order laboratory in one week. He returned to the office in one week. He complained of erectile dysfunction but was otherwise doing well. Laboratory is shown below (Table 7).

Table 7.

	Glucose (mg/dL)	BUN (mg/dL)	Scr (mg/dL)	eGFR (ml/min)	$HbA_1c\%$
Fasting	276	50	3.5	22.4	13.7
2hPP	388	ND	ND	ND	ND

ND = Not done.

Glucose control improved. Renal function still low, still remains anemic. Authors action included 1.) Increase Lantus insulin to 35 units after breakfast and 35 units after dinner and switch Humulin N to Humulin R 20 units before each meal and at bedtime. 2.) Change furosemide to bumetanide 2mg P.O daily 3.) Laboratory in 3 weeks.

Three weeks later, he showed slight edema. Strikingly, he admitted that his vision is improving with insulin therapy. Blood pressure was 145/80. Laboratory is shown in Table 8.

Table 8.

	Glucose (mg/dL)	**BUN (mg/dL)**	**Scr (mg/dL**	**eGFR (ml/min)**	**$HbA_1c\%$**
Fasting	165	52	3.38	23	11.1
2hPP	213	53	3.58	21	ND

Carbon dioxide 20mmol/L.
Uric acid 12.1mg/dL.
CPK units/L 253 high.

Glucose control is rapidly improving characterized by a decrease in fasting and 2h postprandial glucose levels as well as a decrease in hemoglobin A1c. However, he is markedly hyperuricemic and showing low CO_2 level and high CPK, suggesting rhabdomyolysis from use of simvastatin. He was admitted to a local hospital and treated with sodium bicarbonate infusion, detemir, and aspart insulin for control of diabetes, chlorthalidone for control of hypertension and allopurinol for hyperuricemia. After 4 days of intensive therapy he felt happy and in parallel with significant improvement of laboratory findings. Findings are shown in Table 9.

His serum CO_2 is 26mmol/L, calcium is 9.3mg/dL, phosphorus 4.2mg/dL and uric acid decreased to 8.8mg/dL. He was discharged from the hospital and followed in the author's office in 2 weeks.

Table 9.

	Glucose (mg/dL)	BUN (mg/dL)	Scr (mg/dL)	eGFR (ml/min)	24h proteinuria (mg)	Crd (ml/min)
Fasting	102	46	3	23	3539	41.9

Crd = Creatinine clearance.

He returned to the office in 2 weeks. He states he feels well. Slight Edema was noted. Medications consist of Lantus insulin 35 units after breakfast and dinner, Humulin R 20 units before each meal, clonidine 0.2 mg P.O TID, hydralazine 75 mg TID, chlorthalidone 50mg daily, amlodipine 10mg daily, Kcl 10 meQ P.O. TID, simvastatin 10mg daily. Laboratory (Fasting) done on February 9, 2014 showed hemoglobin 9.3g/dL. Glucose 258/mg/dL, serum creatinine 3.34 mg/dL with eGFR 23 ml/min. HbA1c 10.2% and uric acid 7.4 mg/dL. Thus, his diabetes is uncontrolled, renal function is low, CKD stage 4 with slight or no improvement. However, uric acid decreased to near normal level. Allopurinol is decreased to 150mg P.O. daily and simvastatin is discontinued. Novolin R changed to aspart insulin 15 units before each meal and 10 units at bedtime. He will return to office, a laboratory will be done before office visit.

Initiation and Scheduling of Insulin Therapy

Author typically starts Lantus insulin 25 units after breakfast and dinner (12 hours apart). The dosage is increased at an interval of four to 6 weeks until satisfactory glucose control is achieved. Most of them additionally need regular insulin. Preferred regular insulin is Novolin R or Humulin R. Depending on the availability some patients take aspart insulin by a standard sliding scale preceded by obtaining finger stick glucose level. (Table 10)

Table 10.

Finger stick glucose level mg/dL	mmol/L	Novolin R units
150-200	8.3-11.1	4
201-250	11.1-13.8	8
251-300	13.9-16.6	12
301-350	16.7-19.4	16
351-400	19.5-22.2	20

Above 400mg (22.2mmol/L) patient is advised to call primary doctor or author or go to a nearby hospital emergency room to determine the cause of uncontrolled hyperglycemia. In those with difficult to control glycemia, fixed doses of Novolin R or aspart of 15-20 units 15-30 minutes before each meal and at bedtime by sliding scale is prescribed. Author recommends insulin by injection and not by flexpen for less pain. Experiences indicate poor glycemic control in those resorting to pen technique. Also fundamentally, there is no difference between regular insulin and rapid acting insulin such as aspart. A study from United Kingdom showed that glycemic control was actually similar during treatment with human regular insulin (HbA_1c 6.2 ± 0.8%) and insulin lispro (6.0% ± 0.9%) [8].

Uncontrolled hyperglycemia is most commonly due to noncompliance in adhering to a prescribed diet intentionally or otherwise. However, even in the best of circumstances, uncontrolled hyperglycemia could be due to urinary tract infection, flu, or pneumonia in and of itself as well as a result of failure to take prescribed doses of insulin due to the illness. Treatment of these incidental conditions, along with aggressive insulin therapy, help to restore good glycemic control.

As insulin therapy is initiated, oral anti-diabetic drugs are discontinued one to two in each visit until they are all discontinued. Frequent office visits at 4 to 8 week intervals are an integral part of diabetes care to ensure and maintain glycemic control, blood pressure control, renal function control, fluid, electrolyte and acid base control. Compositely, these controls ascertain healthy living and a complication-free life as well as enhancing the ability to cope with the disease and yet thrive [5].

Monitoring of Glycemic Control

There are two ways to monitor day-to-day glucose control. These are 1) finger stick practice using a glucometer and glucose strips 2) urine glucose testing. Although urine glucose testing is simple and cheap, the quantitive assay has not been developed to adjust the insulin dosage based on urine glucose readings. On the other hand, finger stick is painful and expensive, but it is the prevalent method of glucose monitoring at home to adjust insulin dosage. Most patients are educated to check sugar in the morning and night. These random levels may be important to determine glycemic level and adjust insulin dosage ups and downs according to their levels of glucose readings. Author recommends sugar testing 1-2 hours after a meal and bedtime to increase or decrease insulin dosage. If bedtime glucose is high, it will increase further through the night and will lead to nocturia resulting in tiredness in the morning. This is a common feature in uncontrolled diabetes. Author recommends a bedtime dose of regular insulin to minimize nocturia and ensure a restful night. Early morning glycemic surge giving rise to fasting hyperglycemia is not uncommon even in the most compliant patients. It is important to understand that this early morning hyperglycemic surge is conductive to good sleep; whereas an extra dose of insulin at bedtime may increase the risk of hypoglycemia, and waking up in early morning. This nocturnal hypoglycemia may be minimized by eating a bedtime snack consisting of a small sandwich and a glass of milk or juice.

Oral Anti-diabetic Agents

Author prescribes in diet non-compliant or in those with difficult glycemic control one of the two agents 1.) acarbose 2.) pioglitazone

Acarbose is an alpha-glucozidase inhibitor, which competitively inhibits alpha-glucosidase enzymes in the gut that digests dietary starch and sucrose. Another is miglitol. The usual dose is 50mg with each meal. It can be increased to 100mg with each meal. The common side effect is flatulence, which forces some patients to stop taking this drug.

Pioglitazone (Actos®) decreases insulin resistance and increases the insulin sensitivity of adipose tissue, skeletal muscle, and the liver. It takes 6 to 14 weeks to achieve maximum effect. Common side effects include weight gain, fluid retention leading to congestive heart failure. Toxic effect to liver may be seen.

Blood Pressure Control

Briefly, hypertension is controlled using beta blockers, calcium channel blockers, a combination of both, sympathetic inhibitors and in resistant cases, with chlorthalidone. Typically atenolol or metoprolol 50mg PO daily alone or in combination with a second generation dihydrophyridine calcium channel blocker such as amlodipine (Norvasc®) 5 to 10mg daily is prescribed to keep blood pressure under 140/80 mmHg (mean arterial blood pressure of less than 95 mmHHg). In African Americans or in those who are inactive, a central inhibitor such as clonidine 0.1-0.2mg PO BID is prescribed or alpha methyldopa (Aldomet®) 500mg PO BID may be prescribed. In resistant cases of hypertension, chlorthalidone 25 to 50mg PO daily is commonly prescribed.

Author does not prescribe ACEI/ARB drug to any patient and discontinues it, if patients were already taking it at the first visit with the author.

Provocative Data on Renal and Blood Pressure Outcomes in Author's Studies

Forty-six adult diabetes patients: 28 females and 18 males were observed for a period of 14.2 months (1.5-115 months). Diagnosis of diabetes was established by 2-h postprandial glucose of ≥ 200mg/dL (11.1mmol/L) and treated by Glargine or detemir insulin administered after breakfast and dinner, with regular insulin by finger-stick glucose 2-h post meal and bedtime. Blood pressure was controlled with antihypertensive therapy with exclusion of ACEI/ARB drugs. Glucose, serum creatinine and estimated glomerular filtration rate and glycosylated hemoglobin at first and last visits were analyzed in total number of patients and in those with 2-hPPG >< 200mg/dL. The results are shown in Table 11, 12, 13 and Figure 1 and 2.

Glucose at last visit was significantly lower (8.4 ± 0.6mmol/L) than the first visit (10.3 ± 0.7mmol/L) in all patients associated with significantly reduced serum creatinine. No change in eGFR was noted between first and last visits (Table 11). Significant reduction of HbA_1c was found in less than 11.1mmol/L group (Table 12). Blood pressure was normal in both visits in all groups (Table 13). No difference was noted in eGFR between first and last visits. Most of the patients had near normal-to-normal eGFR (Figure 1). Figure 2 reveals recovery of renal function with insulin and discontinuation of oral antidiabetic drugs and ACEI/ARB drugs. Thus, the paradigm of therapy presented here is proven effective in renal preservation in diabetes.

Pearl of Wisdom

1. Define diabetes or diabetes mellitus by obtaining fasting and 2h postprandial (PP) metabolic panel. 2hPP glucose greater than 200mg per dL establishes diabetes.

2. Insulin is the cornerstone of therapy in established diabetes. Insulin is a gift of life for diabetes, it prevents complications and allows subjects to live a healthy life except for a few needle pricks a day.
3. Blood pressure control is an integral part of diabetes therapy, which reduces the risk of complications
4. Avoid use of ACEI/ARB drugs. These drugs have no place in diabetes care.
5. Good glycemic control with insulin reduces proteinuria. Manipulation of proteinuria with ACEI/ARB invariably results in acute renal failure or chronic renal failure with progression to end stage renal disease

Table 11. Average fasting (F), 2 hour Postprandial (2hPP) and d (2hPP-Fasting) glucose, serum creatinine and eGFR at first and last visits in all patients and when 2hPP glucose is > or < 11.1mmol/L

	All patients n=46			>11.1mmol/L n=31			<11.1mmol/L n=15		
Glucose	F	2hPP	d	F	2hPP	d	F	2hPP	d
First visit mmol/L	10.3 ± 0.7	15.2 ± 0.9	5.6 ± 0.6	11.2 ± 0.8	16.1 ± 1.1	5.7 ± 0.7	8.4 ± 1.2	13.5 ± 1.6	5.3 ± 1.2
Last visit mmol/L	8.4 ± 06	14.0 ± 0.8	5.6 ± 0.6	9.6 ± 0.8	16.4 ±0.7	6.7 ± 0.6	5.7 ± 0.3	8.9 ± 0.6	3.3 ± 0.5
*P values	0.017	0.281	0.975	0.124	0.839	0.262	0.048	0.009	0.073
Scr	F	2hPP	d	F	2hPP	d	F	2hPP	d
First visit µmol/L	110.9 ± 7.8	109.4 ± 6.1	6.0 ± 1.3	99.1 ± 7.4	105.6 ± 7.9	6.6 ± 1.6	113.8 ± 8.8	118.5 ± 8.4	4.8 ± 2.3
Last visit µmol/L	100.3 ± 5.2	106.0 ± 5.6	5.8 ± 1.0	95.8 ± 6.3	101.2 ± 6.8	5.4 ± 1.2	111.0 ± 9.2	117.6 ± 9.7	6.6 ± 2.1
*P values	0.013	0.167	0.846	0.214	0.149	0.539	0.552	0.823	0.438
eGFR	F	2hPP	d	F	2hPP	d	F	2hPP	d
First visit mL/min	56.4 ± 2.8	54.7 ± 2.8	-1.61 ± 0.6	59.6 ± 3.4	57.1 ± 3.5	-2.4 ± 0.9	49.7 ± 3.1	48.2 ± 3.2	-3.09 ± 0.09
Last visit mL/min	58.9 ± 3.2	57.0 ± 3.3	-1.94 ± 0.5	60.5 ± 3.4	58.6 ± 3.6	-1.9 ± 0.6	56.2 ± 6.5	53.3 ± 6.4	-2.9 ± 1.10
*P values	0.202	0.257	0.601	0.642	0.494	0.516	0.195	0.262	0.270

Mean ± SEM

*two-tailed paired t-test comparing differences between first and last visits for each parameter.

Table 12. Glycosylated Hemoglobin (HbA_1c) at first and last visits in all patients and when 2hPP Glucose is > or < 11.1 mmol/L

	First visit	Last visit	P values
	HbA_1c%	HbA_1c%	
All patients	9.15 ± 0.32	8.61 ± 0.29	0.1785
> 11.1mmol/L	9.16 ± 0.41	9.12 ± 0.33	0.9356
< 11.1mmol/L	9.14 ± 0.52	7.60 ± 0.45	0.0148

Table 13. Average Systolic, Diastolic and Mean Blood Pressures at first and last visits in all patients and when 2hPP Glucose is > or < 11.1mmol/L

		First visit mmHg	Last visit mmHg	*P values First vs. Last
All patients	Systolic	136.2 ± 3.3	133.6 ± 2.6	0.4777
	Diastolic	81.6 ± 1.9	77.0 ± 1.5	0.297
	Mean	99.8 ± 2.0	77.0 ± 1.5	0.0806
>11.1mmol/L	Systolic	135.7 ± 4.2	133.1 ± 2.7	0.5495
	Diastolic	81.93 ± 2.3	77.6 ± 1.7	0.0795
	Mean	99.9 ± 2.6	96.1 ± 1.4	0.1383
<11.1mmol/L	Systolic	137.2 ± 5.4	134.6 ± 5.8	0.7154
	Diastolic	80.9 ± 3.5	75.7 ± 3.2	0.2233
	Mean	99.9 ± 3.4	95.3 ± 3.4	0.3644

* two-tailed paired t-test.

References

[1] Frederick Banting Nobel Prize speech September 15, 1925 In *History of Diabetes Mellitus Elsevier Masson* 2009 Page 49-62.

[2] Willis Hurst J, What do good doctors try to do? *Commentary Arch Interm Med* 2003; 163: 2681-2686.

[3] Mandal AK, Puchalski JT, Lemley-Gillespie S, Taylor CA, and Kohno M. Effect of insulin and heparin on glucose-induced vascular damage in cell culture. *Kidney Int* 2000; 57: 2492-2501.

[4] Fabre J, Balant LP, Dayer PG, Fox HM, and Vernet AT: Kidney in mature onset diabetes mellitus: a clinical study of 510 patients. *Kidney Int* 1982; 21: 730-738.

[5] Mandal AK, Frequent office visits of patients with chronic kidney disease: Is a prelude to prevention of dialysis. *World Journal of Nephrology* 2014; 3: 1-5.

[6] Saydah SH, Miret M, Sung J, Varas C, Gause O, Brancate FL Post challenge hyperglycemia and mortality in national sample of US adults, *Diab Care* 2001; 26: 1397-1402.

[7] Gerich JE Clinical significance, pathogenesis and management of postprandial hyperglycemia. *Arch Intern Med* 2003; 163: 1306-16.

[8] Heller SR, Amiel SA, Mansell F, UK Lispro study Group. Effect of fast acting insulin analog lispro on the risk of nocturnal hypoglycemia during intensified insulin therapy. *Diab Care* 1999; 22: 1607-1611.

Chapter X

Obesity with Type 2 Diabetes Is a Surrogate of Metabolic Syndrome

Abstract

Obesity is steadily increasing in the society since the end of World War II, and followed by economic development, greater availability of consumable products and sedentary lifestyle. Obesity is frequently associated with impaired glucose tolerance mimicking diabetes with 2-h postprandial glucose level ≥ 200mg/dL (≥ 11.1mmol/L). This hyperglycemia is connoted as Type 2 diabetes mellitus (T2DM). Since the hyperglycemia or so-called T2DM undergoes resolution because of massive weight loss following bariatric surgery, a strong argument can be made that T2DM is not the same as diabetes due to insulin deficiency as defined by Frederick Banting in 1925. Diabetes undergoes remission but insulin levels do not change. Literature is filled with information on gut-derived hormones such as incretins as a mechanism for weight reduction and remission of T2DM. Sometimes reversal of T2DM occurs even before significant weight loss has occurred thereby supporting incretin theory and or another gut hormone called Ghelin. Ghelin stimulates appetite and is decreased markedly following Roux-en-y gastric bypass surgery. Although much is published about incretin, no evidence is available on the pathophysiological correlation between weight reduction, incretin levels, and remission of type 2 diabetes. Thus, it is prudent to state that the actual mechanism leading to diabetes resolution following bariatric surgery remains to be elucidated.

Introduction

The prevalence of obesity has increased steadily since ending World War II, followed by economic development, greater availability of consumable products and sedentary life style. Currently, more than 10% of the world's adult population is obese, as determined by a body mass index (BMI) equal to or greater than 30Kg/m^2. In the USA, the prevalence of obesity is 34%. Obesity is caused by an imbalance between intake and expenditure of energy and is particularly associated with increased adiposity. Obesity is frequently associated with impaired glucose tolerance mimicking diabetes with 2h postprandial glucose level of ≥200mg/dL (≥11.1mmol/L). This hyperglycemia is connoted as Type 2 diabetes mellitus (T2 DM). However, this hyperglycemia may not be same as diabetes defined by insulin deficiency. The connotation of Type 2 DM in obese individuals is a misnomer. As it will be found here later, hyperglycemia or so called Type 2 DM remits because of massive weight loss following bariatric surgery. A 4-hour oral glucose tolerance test will disprove prior existence of diabetes, which undergoes resolution because of weight loss in obese individuals. All these will unfold later in this chapter. Let us find out the relationship between obesity and hyperglycemia.

Obesity can lead to impairment of insulin sensitivity in sites of glucose disposal, such as skeletal muscle, liver, and adipose tissue – a condition known as "insulin resistance." The normal action of insulin includes stimulation of glucose uptake and glycogen synthesis in the skeletal muscles and liver and inhibition of neoglucogenesis in the liver. Insulin also causes inhibition of lipolysis and increases lipogenesis in adipose tissue. Insulin resistance is characterized by reduced glucose uptake by skeletal muscles, increased release of glucose from the liver and increased release of lipids from adipose tissue into the blood. Overall, all these result in glucose intolerance and unabated hyperglycemia despite high doses of insulin without or with use of oral antidiabetic agents in obese individuals. It has been stated repeatedly in the literature that compensatory hyper-secretion of insulin can lead to beta cell failure and eventual development of overt diabetes [1].

Again it will be found in the section of case report that with massive weight loss hyperglycemia remits spontaneously and a normal glucose challenge test will disprove diabetes in obese individuals after weight loss. A study from Morocco is testimonial to the existence of metabolic syndrome. Moroccan scientists have reported that rapid Moroccan economic growth in recent decades has created drastic changes in the lifestyle of the Moroccan population. Excess energy intake and sedentary life style is becoming widespread in the population, and increasing metabolic risk factors such as obesity, diabetes, and hypertension to the epidemic level. Metabolic syndrome is a group of inter-related risk factors of metabolic origin that appear to directly promote the development of atherosclerotic cardiovascular disease and Type 2 DM [2].

Case Reports of Obesity and Diabetes

Patient #1

A 53-year-old white male was first seen by the author in August 2010. He gave a history of diabetes of ten to twelve years in duration. He fell and went to the emergency room of a local hospital and was found to have diabetes. Significantly, he was not active and he has experienced erectile dysfunction. He stated that home finger stick glucose levels varied between 100 and 200mg/dL but sometimes jumped to over 400mg/dL. His legs go to sleep and experienced tingling and numbness in the feet. Past history included follow up in different clinics since year 2002 apparently for diabetes but no laboratory information is available to document diabetes. Family history of diabetes was not known to the patient. Physical examination: weight 338lbs, pulse 112 beats/min, regular, blood pressure sitting 150/70 mmHg and upright 170/70 mmHg. Slight edema was noted in the lower extremity bilaterally. Heart sounds were normal and a few rales were heard on chest auscultation. Medications consisted of glyburide/metformin 5/500mg 2 tablets twice daily, levothyroxine 200mcg daily, amlodipine 5mg daily, lisinopril 20mg daily, gemfibrozil 600mg twice daily, crestor 10mg daily, tamsulosin 0.4mg daily, triamterene-hydrochlorothiazide 37.5/25mg once daily, prevacid 30mg daily, Isosorbide 30mg daily. He had a laboratory done in March 2010, which showed HbA_1c 5.9%, hemoglobin 16.3g/dL and hematocrit 47.6%. A urinalysis was negative. He was prescribed atenolol 50mg daily and basic metabolic panel (Fasting and 2h postprandial), serum insulin, and TSH were ordered. 1600 calories ADA diet was advised. He returned in one month. His weight decreased to 333lbs and sitting blood pressure decreased to 100/60mmHg. His fasting glucose was 90mg/dL and 2hPP glucose 120mg/dL, average glucose was 177mg/dL and HbA_1c was 7.8%. Renal function was normal, eGFR was 101.1ml/min. Serum insulin level (2h postprandial) was 36.1 mclU/ml (N= 2.6-24.9 mcIU/ml). At this visit, lisinopril and triam/hydrochlorthiazide (HCTZ) were discontinued. He returned to the office 3 months later. His blood pressure increased to sitting 180/100mmHg. His fasting and 2hPP glucose levels were 131mg/dL and 181mg/dL, respectively. HbA_1c was 8.4%. Medications were adjusted, and triam/HCTZ was resumed for hypertension. In December 2010, his blood pressure was normal but both fasting (FBG) and 2hPP glucose (2hPPG) increased to 236mg/dL and 267mg/dL, respectively. HbA_1c increased to 9.2% and urinalysis showed 1+ protein. He was started on glargine insulin (Lantus) after breakfast and dinner, and Novolin R with each meal and at bed time. Triam/HCTZ was reduced from daily dosing to Mondays and Fridays only. One month later, his glucose levels decreased but HbA_1c remained unchanged. In March 2011, his glucose levels were slightly elevated but hemoglobin HbA_1c decreased. By June 2011, his weight increased to 341lbs, his glucose levels and HbA_1c are slightly elevated with normal renal function. He was treated with glargine insulin and Novolin R. His weight kept increasing and reached 350lbs in October 2011, postprandial hyperglycemia persisted despite high dose of insulin. Bariatric surgery was recommended. A Roux-en-y gastric bypass surgery was done in November 2011. In this surgery, a gastric pouch is created that completely separates the gastric remnant and is anastomosed to the jejunum. The gastric pouch restricts food intake. The bypass of the duodenum and part of the jejunum reduces absorption. Immediately following surgery all three glycemic parameters including FBG, 2hPPG and HbA_1c are all normal. Insulin was discontinued. He only takes atenolol 50mg daily and amlodipine 10mg daily to keep his blood pressure under control. His most recent visit was on January 2015. His sitting blood pressure was 80/40mmHg and pulse 58/min. Atenolol was discontinued. Later part of 2013, a urinalysis showed many hyaline casts which raised the suspicion of glomerular disease. A hepatitis profile showed reactive hepatitis C. A percutaneous kidney biopsy was done not to document diabetes change but to determine if he has developed membranous or membranoproliferative glomerulonephritis (GN). To a total surprise kidney biopsy showed severe arteriolar hyalinosis and mild to moderate arteriosclerosis. Focal tubulointerstitial nephritis was noted. There was no evidence of diabetic glomerulosclerosis or immune complex glomerulonephritis GN (Figure 1-3)

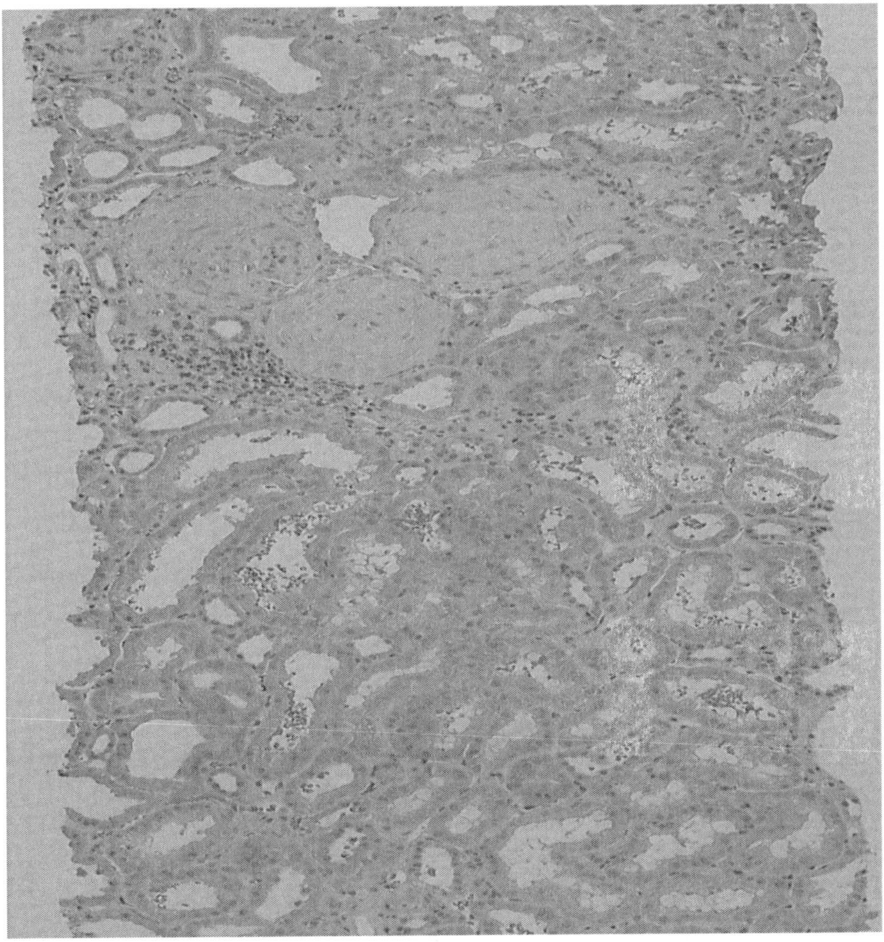

Figure 1. Kidney biopsy shows arterialor hyalinosis and normal tubules. Light microscopy (Hematoxyllin and cosin).

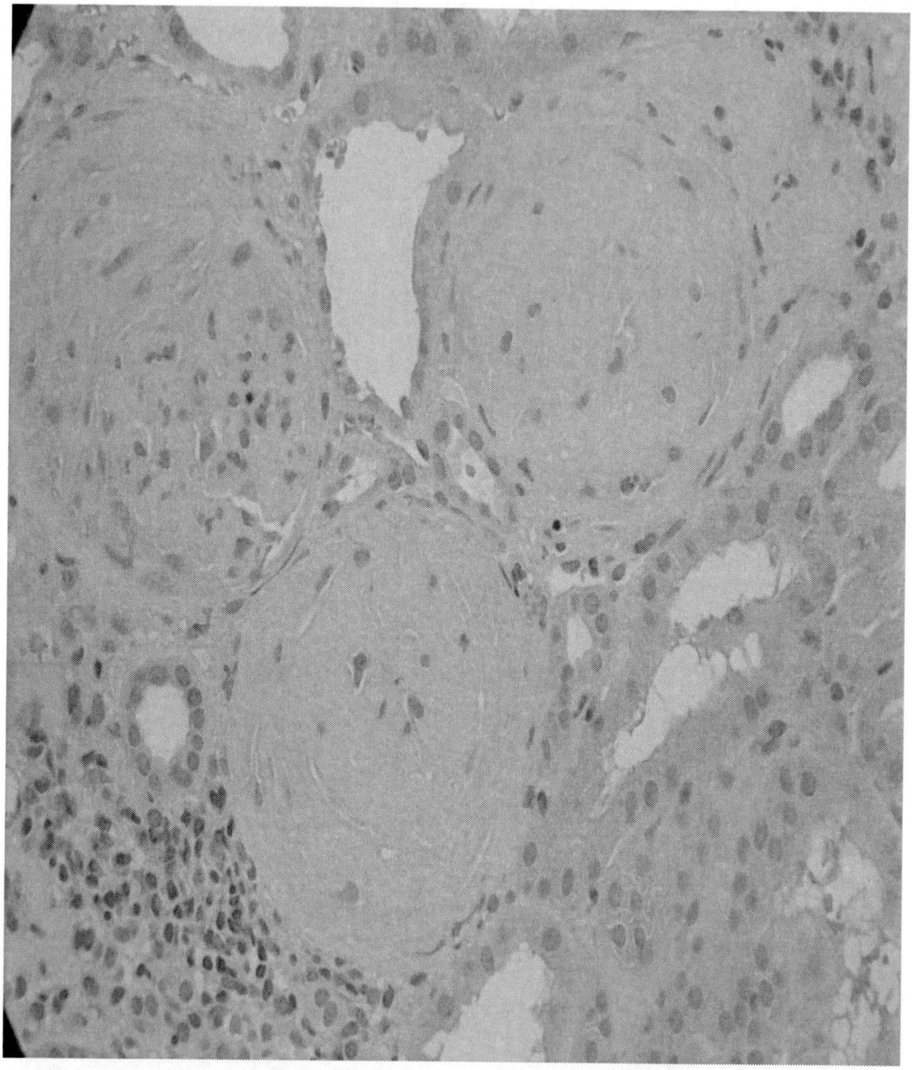

Figure 2. High power view of arteriolar hyalinosis. Light microscopy (Hematoxylin and cosin).

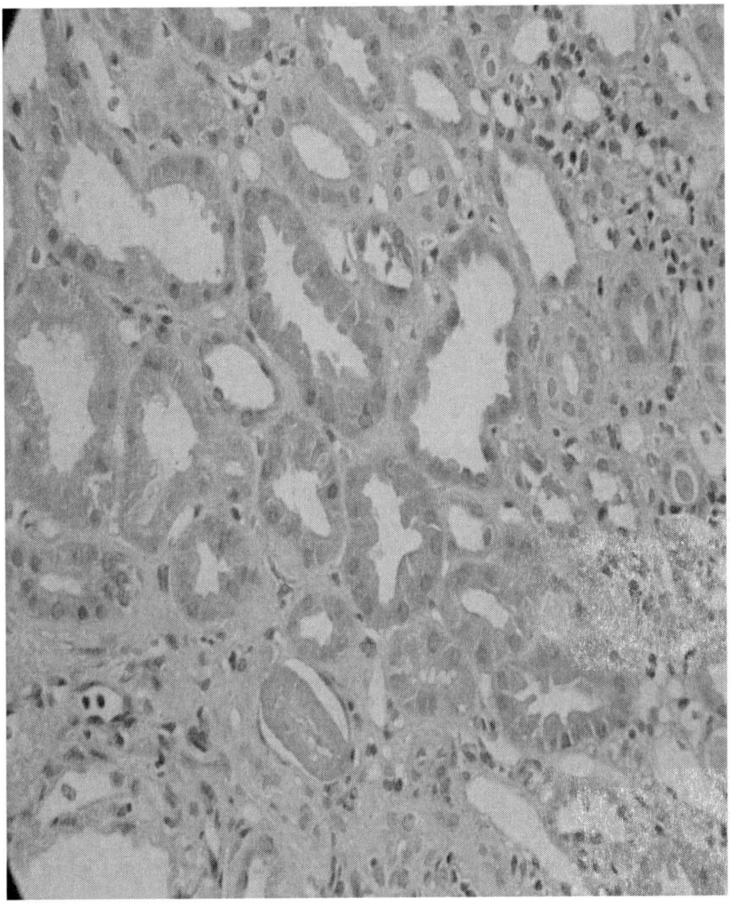

Figure 3. A portion of kidney biopsy showing normal appearing tubules with a few cellular infiltrate on the right. Light microscopy (Hematoxylin and cosin).

He did a 4-h oral glucose tolerance in December 2014. The results are shown below.

4-h Glucose Tolerance Test

Fasting	52mg/dL (2.8mmol/L)
1 hour	107mg/dL (5.9mmol/L)
2 hour	65mg/dL (3.6mmol/L)
3 hour	93mg/dL (5.1mmol/L)
4 hour	82mg/dL (4.5mmol/L)

Fasting hypoglycemia is noted. Glucose levels from 1-4 hours are lower than normal. His appetite is good but he can eat only small portions. His medications consist of atenolol 50mg daily, amlodipine 10mg daily, and pentoxifylline 400mg PO TID, and levothyroxine 225mcg daily. His sitting blood pressure is 120/80mmHg. His most recent laboratory results in 2015 are shown below:

	Glucose mg/dL(mmol/L)	**Scr (mg/dL)**	**eGFR ml/min**	**HbA_1c% Avg glucose mg/dL**	**Serum insulin Mc IU/ml**	**Serum cortisol Mcg/dL**
Fasting	89 (4.9)	0.52	>110	5.5/111	13.3	18.4
2hPP	126 (7)	0.50	>110	ND	27.4*	26.5

* Ref Range 2.6 - 24.9.
ND = Not done.

Thus, his glucose levels and HbA_1c are normal. His insulin responses are appropriate. His cortisol levels are normal. All these glycemic levels and insulin responses three years and 2 months after bariatric surgery should be attributed to resolution of diabetes and not a remission of diabetes. Thus if this patient is seen by another doctor without knowing that he had gastric bypass surgery, that doctor will qualify him as a normal subject.

Patient #2

A 51-year-old white female with morbid obesity, weighing 301 pounds, was first seen in the office in March 2010 referred by a primary care physician for control of uncontrolled diabetes, and treatment of hypokalemia and hypomagnesemia. She had a bilateral knee replacement left and right in 2005 and 2006, respectively. Her main complaint was a problem with uncontrolled diabetes for several years. She also gave a history of hypertension for 2 to 3 years. Past history was significant for hospital admission for chest pain but no abnormality was detected in the heart. She underwent total hysterectomy for heavy menstrual bleeding. She has no children. She does not smoke or drink alcohol. Medications at this visit consisted of repaglinide 1mg TID before meal, glipizide 10mg BID, furosemide 40mg daily, Januvia 100mg daily, simvastatin 40mg at bed time, potassium chloride 10mEq X 2 BID, magnesium oxide 400mg BID. She was advised to take insulin but she was afraid of injections. Laboratory on March 1, 2010 (Random) showed glucose 254mg/dL, serum Na 141mmol/L, serum K 3.4mmol/L, serum creatinine

1.07mg/dL and eGFR of 58ml/min. Serum magnesium was 1.4mg/dL. At this visit, repaglinide and furosemide were discontinued. She was advised to resort to 1600 calories ADA diet. She was hospitalized in early May 2010 for control of diabetes and started on glargine insulin 25 units after breakfast and dinner. She was also started on metformin 500mg twice daily and started on clonidine 0.1mg twice daily and hydrochlorothiazide 12.5mg daily for blood pressure control. She was seen in the office on May 27, 2010. Her sitting blood pressure was 160/60mmHg. Laboratory (fasting) showed glucose 158mg/dL, serum Na and K of 137/3.8 mmol/L, respectively, serum creatinine 0.77mg/dL and eGFR 60ml/min. She was lost for follow up and came back for an office visit two years later. Her main complaint was swelling of legs. Therapy was essentially same except Kcl was substituted by spironolactone 50mg twice daily. Laboratory (fasting) showed glucose 147mg/dL, essentially unchanged renal function and low magnesium of 1.3mg/dL. She was prescribed magnesium oxide 400mg PO TID.

She had an office visit on June 1, 2012 with fasting and 2h postprandial (2hPP) basic metabolic panel (BMP) done. Also, she had urinalysis done and insulin levels at fasting and 2h postprandial period. Results are shown in the table below

	Glucose mg/dL/mmol/L	**Scr (mg/dL)**	**eGFR (ml/min)**	**K (mmol/L)**	**Insulin Mclu/ml**
Fasting	202/11.2	1.14	53	4.6	15.9
2hPP	229/12.7	1.21	49	4.7	24.9

Scr = serum creatinine.
K= Potassium.
*Ref range 2.6 – 24.9.

At this visit, glargine insulin increased to 35 units after breakfast and 35 units after dinner. Metformin was discontinued. She also was advised not to take spironolactone because of increased serum potassium. She was registered for gastric bypass surgery. To that effect, a percutaneous kidney biopsy was done to determine the extent of diabetic nephropathy in March 2014. Light microscopy of the kidney biopsy showed diffuse and nodular glomerulosclerosis (Figure 1 and Figure 2). Moderate arterial and arteriolar sclerosis with hyalinosis was noted (Figure 2) Nodular glomerulosclerosis is evident but tubules anatomically appeared normal (Figure 3).

At this point of time, she was treated with insulin detemir (Levemir®) 70 units after breakfast and 70 units after dinner and lispro insulin (Humalog®) 35 units before each meal and at bedtime. She was restarted on metformin

1000mg twice daily. She was taking clonidine and amlodipine for blood pressure control. Her sitting blood pressure was normal 120/60mmHg. Her F and 2hPP BMP are shown in the table below.

	Glucose mg/dL (mmol/L)	**Scr (mg/dL)**	**eGFR (ml/min)**	**U Protein**	**Serum Albumin (g/dL)**
Fasting	205	0.90	>60	1+	3.2
2hPP	269	0.95	>60	ND	ND

Scr= serum creatinine; U protein= urine; ND= Not done.

During this visit, acarbose 100mg PO with each meal was prescribed.

In subsequent office visits in 2014, glycemia control could not be achieved but kidney function has remained normal. She didn't go for bariatric surgery.

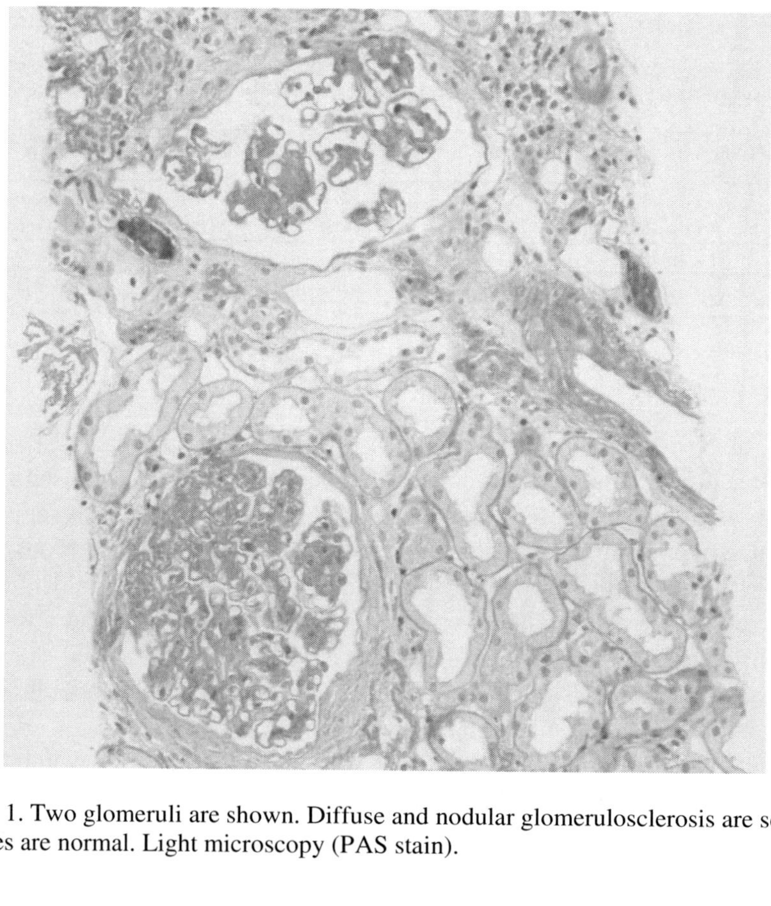

Figure 1. Two glomeruli are shown. Diffuse and nodular glomerulosclerosis are seen. Tubules are normal. Light microscopy (PAS stain).

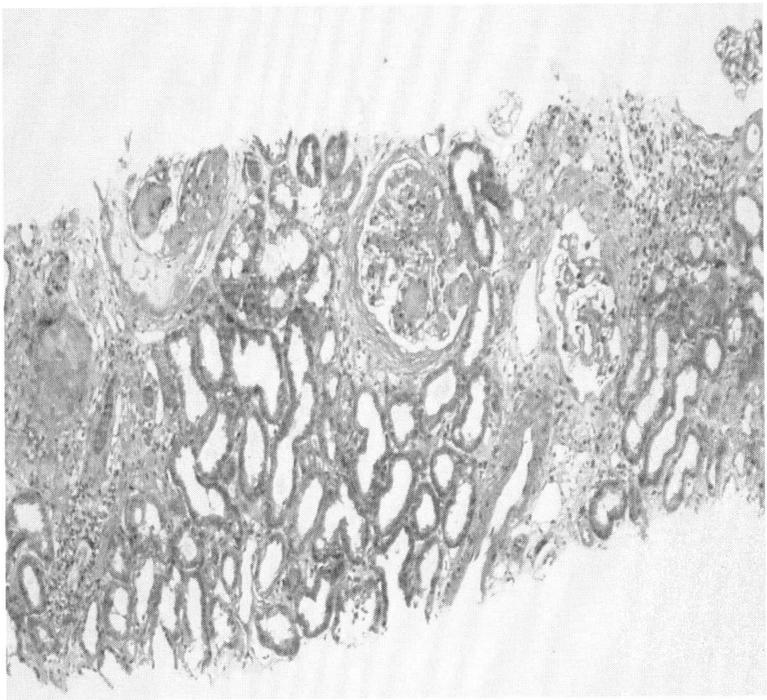

Figure 2. Two glomeruli are seen. Both show nodular glomerulosclerosis. To the left of glomeruli arteriolar hyalinosis is seen. Light microscopy (PAS stain).

Impact of Massive Weight Reduction on Renal Pathology Associated with Diabetes

Both patients presented here are obese, one with more obesity than the other. Patient number one underwent Roux-en-y gastric bypass surgery but patient number two refused the procedure. Patient number one represents a unique example of resolution of metabolic problem in addition to reduction of weight of 125 pounds following bariatric surgery. Metabolic response was immediate. All glycemic parameters including fasting glucose (FBG), 2 hour postprandial glucose (2hPPG), and glycosylated hemoglobin (HbA_1c) were all normal and requiring no insulin within a month following bariatric surgery. Two years following bariatric surgery, a kidney biopsy showed no evidence of diabetic nephropathoy. Arteriolar hyalinosis observed in kidney biopsy specimen may be telltale evidence of diabetic nephropathy. Considering that possibility, it may be surmised that he had diabetic nephropathy, which had undergone resolution in parallel with resolution of metabolic abnormalities following bariatric surgery. Comparing this patient with patient number two, who is equally obese but refused bariatric surgery, shows uncontrolled diabetes despite high doses of a combination of detemir and fast acting insulin. Her kidney biopsy showed diffuse and nodular diabetic glomerulosclerosis but minimal tubulointerstitial changes. Her renal function tests are normal. These two disparate renal pathologies, with and without bariatric surgery, respectively, raise an important question, which is one of the two: weight reduction or surgery in and of itself makes the outcome difference.

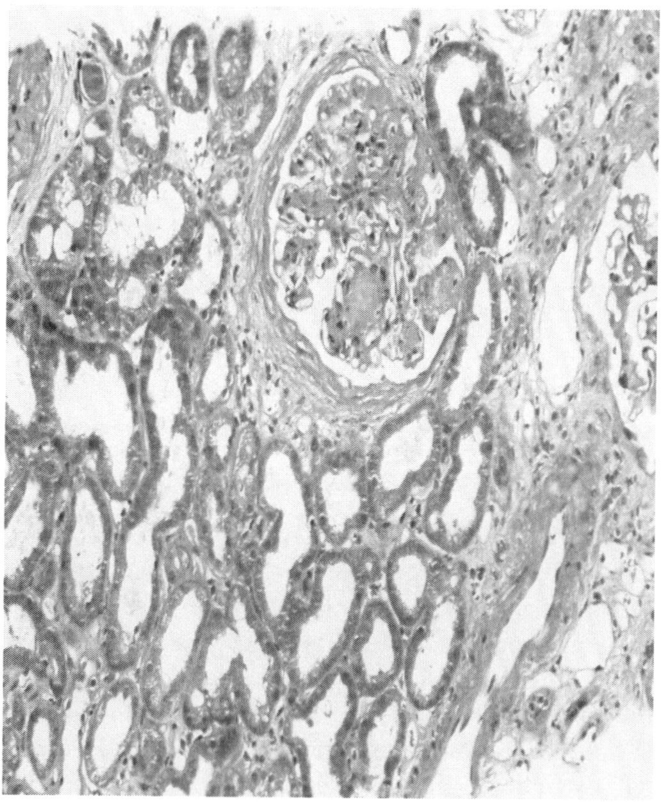

Figure 3. A high power view of a glomerulus showing nodular glomerulosclerosis at 12 o'clock position typical of kimmelsteil-wilson syndrome – a forgotten syndrome. Tubules are normal. Light microscopy (PAS stain).

Effect of Bariatric Surgery on the Mechanism of Resolution of Diabetes

Review of literature reveals remission of diabetes [3, 4] following bariatric surgery but no information is available about how the remission was defined. In one article, remission was defined as fasting blood glucose levels lower than 110mg/dL and no diabetic medication. No mechanism for remission of diabetes was stated. We concur with the pathogenesis of postprandial hyperglycemia by Lebovitz [5]. Muscle glucose uptake is the major mechanism by which postprandial plasma glucose is cleared. Thus, the earliest abnormality of intermediary metabolism that occurs in diabetes is postprandial hyperglycemia. The difference in postprandial hyperglycemia before and after bariatric surgery will confirm that. Patient number one had ten times FBG and 2hPPG and nine times HbA_1c drawn before bariatric surgery; and seventeen times FBG and 2hPPG and eleven times HbA_1c drawn after bariatric surgery. The results are shown in the next table.

	FBG mg/dL (mmol/L)	**2hPPG mg/dL**	**HbA_1c%**
Before bariatric surgery	142 (7.8)	198 (11mmol/L)	8.3
After bariatric surgery	109.9 (6.1)	104.8 (5.8)	5.6

Sustained mean 2h postprandial glucose (2hPPG) higher than fasting glucose (FBG) before bariatric surgery and 2hPPG lower than FBG after bariatric surgery is a testimony of better clearing of 2hPPG by muscle, with marked loss of weight.

Literature is filled with information on gut-derived hormones as a mechanism for weight reduction and remission of diabetes [6, 7]. Incretins are gut-derived hormones that stimulate insulin production. Glucagon-like peptide (GLP-1) and gastric inhibitory peptide (GIP) are the important and most studied incretins. Following RYGB increases in plasma concentrations of the incretin hormone GLP-1 have been recorded and the known antidiabetic effects of GLP-1 are thought to be the key mediators in RYGB-induced remission of T2DM. However, the published studies on the impact of RYGB on GLP-1 secretion are few, small and without clinicopathological correlation [7]. An increased GLP-1 concentration after RYGB may be caused by delivery of nutrients to the distal ileum. Sometimes diabetes reversal occurs even before significant weight loss has occurred, which may be attributed to incretin theory and or another gut hormone called Ghelin. Ghelin is produced in the stomach and duodenum; it stimulates appetite. Ghelin levels decrease substantially after RYGB [6]. A previous study has provided a review of the possible underlying mechanisms leading to resolution of Type 2 diabetes symptoms after RYGB procedure. The actual mechanism leading to diabetes resolution remains unknown [8].

References

[1] Wali JA, Thomas HE, Sutherland APR Liking obesity with Type 2 diabetes: the role of T-bet Diab, Metab Syndrome and Obesity; *Target and Therapy* 2014; 7: 331-340.

[2] Elbirini O, Akhouayri O, Gamal A, Mesfiouri A, Benazzouz B Prevalence of metabolic syndrome and its components based on harmonious definition among adults in Morocco Diab Met Syndrome and Obesity: *Target and Therapy* 2014; 7: 341-346.

[3] Dixon JB, Zimmet P, Alberti G et al. Bariatric surgery for diabetes: The international diabetes federation takes a position *J Diabetes* 2011; 3: 261-264.

[4] Sjostrom L, Peltonen M, Jacobson P et al. Association of bariatric surgery with long-term remission of Type 2 diabetes and with microvascular and macrovascular complications *JAMA* 2014; 311: 2297-2303.

[5] Lebovitz HE Postprandial hyperglycemic state: Importance and consequences *Diab Res clinPract* 1998; 40: 527-528.

[6] Meijer RI, Van Wagensveld BA, Stegert CE et al. Bariatric Surgery as novel treatment for Type 2 diabetes mellitus *Arch Surg* 2011; 146: 744-750.

[7] Rhee NA, Vilsboll T, Knop FK Bypass-induced remission of Type 2 diabetes *J AmcollSurg* 2012; 214: 550-6.

[8] Lee TI, Chen JH, Weng TC et al. Gastric bypass and diabetes: past, present and future. *Curr Diabetes Rev* 2011; 7 (5) 305-12.

Chapter XI

Role of Self-care in Management of Diabetes Mellitus

Abstract

The management of diabetes mellitus (DM) consists of glycemic control with insulin therapy with a goal to reduce the risk of development or progression of diabetic complications. Most of the diabetic complications are disabling and very costly to treat. Thus, prevention is fundamentally important. Understanding the illness and taking responsibility of the illness can go a long way to prevent the disabling complications. There are several self-care behaviors in people with diabetes that predict good outcomes, namely prescribed diabetic diet, physical activity, home monitoring of blood sugar, taking prescribed doses of insulin and the ability to cope with illness and thrive. All these behaviors have been found to be positively correlated with good glycemic control, reduction of complications and improvement in quality of life. Despite the value of these behaviors, long-term adherence to these behaviors varies. Some are very adherent while others are not, especially when understanding of the severity of the illness is poor. Here comes counseling by the professionals who can turn patients around and increase their adherence to daily routine.

Introduction

Diabetes mellitus (DM) is characterized by insulin deficiency or slow response to glucose challenge and associated with hyperglycemia in excess of 200mg/dL (11.1mmol/L) in an untreated state and variable amounts of glycosuria. DM virtually affects every system of the body mainly due to high glucose milieu especially when glucose control is inadequate.

Untreated or uncontrolled diabetes gives rise to a gamut of complications such as coronary artery disease, neuropathy, nephropathy, retinopathy, sexual dysfunction and neurogenic bladder; all of these give rise to high morbidity and mortality. Almost 80% of diabetes deaths occur in low and middle-income countries. Recent surveys indicate that diabetes now affects a staggering 10-16% of the urban population and 5-8% of the rural population in India and Sri Lanka.

Needs of Patients with Diabetes

Previous studies have reported that strict metabolic control can delay or prevent progression of complications associated with diabetes [1, 2]. The needs of diabetic patients are not only limited to adequate glycemic control but also intended to prevention of complications and disabilities.

Some of the Indian studies reveal very poor adherence to treatment regimens due to poor attitude toward the disease and poor health literacy among the general public. The introduction of home blood glucose monitors and widespread use of glycosylated hemoglobin as an indicator of metabolic control has contributed to self-care in diabetes and this has shifted more responsibility to the patients.

Self-care in Diabetes

In a study done in Scotland, it was suggested that the role of the health professionals is crucial to patient's understanding of their blood glucose fluctuation with appropriate self-care actions [3].

Self-care in diabetes has been defined as an evolutionary process of development of knowledge or awareness by learning to thrive and cope with the complex nature of the illness. Because the vast majority of day-to-day care in diabetes is handled by patients and or families, there is an important need for reliable and valid measures for self-management of diabetes. There are seven essential self-care behaviors in people with diabetes, which predict good outcomes. These are adherence to prescribed diabetic diet, stay active, do finger stick glucose, in particular 2 hours post meal and bedtime, take prescribed dose of insulin, learn to cope with the illness and stay optimistic to live a good life with good control of diabetes. All these behaviors have been found to be positively correlated with good glycemic control, reduction of complications and improvement in quality of life. In addition, it was observed that self-care encompasses not only performing these activities but also determining the inter-relationship between them. Diabetes self-care requires the patients to make dietary and life-style modifications supplemented with the supportive role of health care staff for maintaining a higher level of self-confidence leading to a behavior change.

Diabetes Self Management Education

Patients with diabetes should educate themselves about the disease process. The more educated they are, the more consistent the self-care will be. It is expected that those with the greatest knowledge will have a better understanding of the disease and have a greater impact on the prevention of progression of the disease or development of its complications. The American Diabetes Association had reviewed the standards of diabetes self-management education and found that there was a four-fold increase in diabetic complications for those individuals with diabetes who had not received formal education concerning self-care practices. However, the observed benefit declined 1 to 3 months after the intervention ceased, suggesting that continuing education should be in place. A review of diabetes self-management education revealed that education is successful in lowering glycosylated hemoglobin [4].

Diabetes Self-care activities and Adherence to Self-care Activities

Diabetes usually requires substantial life-long self-management by the patient. Psychological factors and the patient's health beliefs are important determinants of self-care behavior. Education has a modest influence in generating better self-care, but psychologically based interventions are more effective.

The diagnosis of diabetes has a major psychological impact. Good glycemic control of diabetes leading to a good long-term medical outcome requires a considerable degree of self-management by the patient. As clinicians we advise patients to undertake a series of self-management tasks: diet and exercise; regular therapy; injections; self-monitoring; self-adjustment of the treatment and clinic visits. The motivation to undertake these behaviors can be limited in a condition where there is little in the way of symptoms. The diagnosis of diabetes has a major psychological impact. Adjustment of the individual to this psychological blow is critical. A major challenge for health care professionals is to support and optimize coping behavior. The provision of education is important in that patients need to know what they need to do.

Empowerment

Patients have to make their own decisions about their diabetes management day to day without professional immediately at hand. The empowerment philosophy emphasizes that patients need the psychosocial skills to achieve behavior change, changes in their social situation, and other factors that influence their lives. Patients need to understand and accept that day to day care of their diabetes is their responsibility with insulin-treated patients, training to adjust their own insulin dose for meal size, fasting or corrections of hyperglycemic control as expected, but also generated greater perceptions of self-efficacy and a feeling of empowerment. Research using self-regulatory theory indicates that personal control is an important part of the patient's personal model of their diabetes. Personal control relates to glycemic control. Empowerment increases the individual's personal control and is therefore consistent with theory [5].

Barriers to Diabetes Care and Recommendation for Self Care Activities

Injectable treatment such as insulin treatment is a fundamental therapy for established diabetes (2h postprandial ≥ 200mg/dL (11.1 mmol/L). Numerous barriers lead to delay in initiating injectable treatment, which in turn may lead to inadequate glycemic control and increased risk of diabetes-related complications. It is needless to underscore the need to understand and address these barriers. Barriers to the initiation of injectable therapy originate from both patients and practitioners. Anxiety about fear of injection-associated pain has been estimated to affect approximately 30%-50% of patients before the initiation of diabetes education interventions. Advances in needle design have minimized the pain associated with injections, and recent data suggests that actual pain and bleeding are associated with various needle gauges (21-gauge to 31-gauge) are mild [6].

Negative perceptions of injectable therapy from patients may stem from familiarity with family members or friends with diabetes who were receiving injectable therapies and went on to experience complications.

In a survey of 501 patients with diabetes who used a syringe or a pen device to deliver insulin, almost half reported injection-related bruising and 37% reported injection-related pain.

It is widely considered that needle length is likely to be associated with increased injection pain, and although there are data that support this view, not all studies are confirmatory. An open-label cross over study of obese patients with diabetes assessed pain with both short (5mm) and long (8mm) needles of the same gauge using a visual analog scale (VAS). The VAS is a linear scale used to assess pain encompassing a range of numbers (0-10 or 1-100) such that the lowest number is indicative of no pain and the highest number is indicative of the worst pain possible. Both needles were associated with low mean VAS scores for pain. With an overall rating of 7 (5mm needle) versus a rating of 9 (8mm needle) out of 100, the difference between the two was not significant (Figure 1). Generally, patients prefer shorter thinner needles, for instance a 6mm needle. With regard to recommendations to improve self-care activities, patients are disappointed to find out for themselves that many health care providers are not discussing self-care activities with their patients. Some patients may experience difficulty in understanding and following the basics of diabetes self-care activities. It is critical that health care providers actively involve their patients in developing self-care regimens for each individual patient. Also the need for regular follow up can never be underestimated in a chronic illness like diabetes, and therefore must be looked upon as an integral component of its long-term management [7].

Pearl of Wisdom

Dedicated self care including diabetes diet, physical activity, treatment with insulin, control of blood pressure with drugs that have no adverse effect on the kidneys will go a long way to reduce morbidity and mortality. Finger stick practices to monitor glucose levels and adjust insulin dosage are essential and permissible for an active and healthy life. It is important to consult health care providers as often as necessary for questions related to finger stick glucose, insulin dosage, episodes of hypoglycemia and change in blood pressure control.

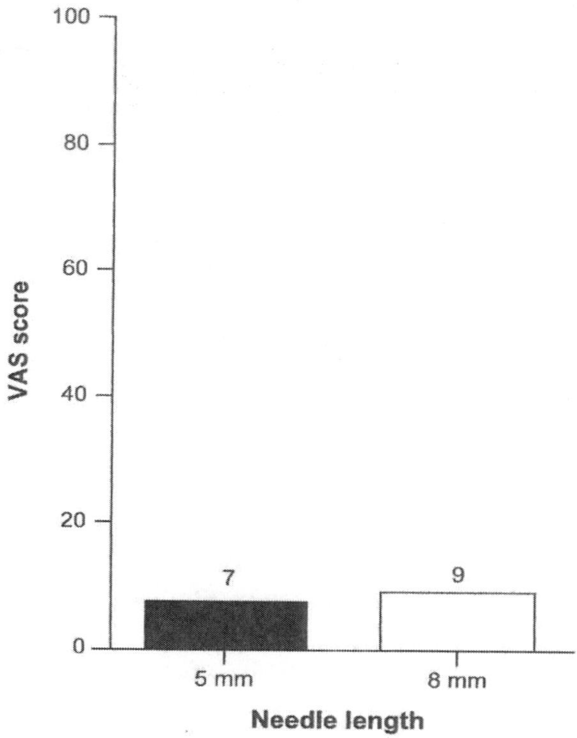

Figure 1. VAS (Visual Analog Scale) pain score for 5mm and 8 mm needles Reproduced with permission.

References

[1] UKPDS Intensive blood glucose control with sulphonylurean or insulin compared with conventional treatment and risk of complications in patients with type 2 diabetes. *Lancet* 1998; 352: 837-853.

[2] Ohkuboy, Kishikanra H, Araki E et al. Intensive insulin therapy prevents the progression of diabetic micro-vascular complications in Japanese patients with non-insulin dependent diabetes mellitus: a randomized prospective 6-year study *Diab Res clin Pract* 1995: 28: 103-117.

[3] Peel E, Douglas M, Lawton J Self monitoring of blood glucose in type 2 diabetes: longitudinal qualitative study of patients perspectives *BMJ* 2007: 335: 493.

[4] Glasgow RE, Strycke LA Preventive care practives for diabetes management in two primary care samples *Am J Prev Med* 2000; 19: 9-14.

[5] Harvey JN Psychosocial interventions for the diabetic patient Diab Met syndrome and obesity; *Targets and therapy* 2015; 8: 29-43.

[6] Kruger DF, LaRue S, Estepa P Recognition and steps to mitigate anxiety and fear of pain in injectable diabetes treatment. Diab Met Syndrome and obesity: *Targets and therapy* 2015; 8: 49-56.

[7] Mandal AK. Frequent office visits of patients with Chronic Kidney disease: Is a prelude to prevention of dialysis. *World J Nephrol* 2014; 3: 1-5.

Index

D

E

F

G

H

I

J

K

L

R

S

T

U

V

W